PREFACE

Question Your Beliefs

In 2017, in a country known for its universal health care coverage, a doctor had his license suspended for treating Lyme patients according to clinical guidelines that meet internationally accepted standards. As a result, currently there are no known doctors in Sweden who are trained in these clinical therapies. Meanwhile, an eight-year-old Swedish boy has been losing more of his ability to talk since he twice tested positive for Lyme borreliosis infection in his nervous system. He was given a short course of antibiotics by his non-Lyme trained physician, and his parents were told not to worry about his increasing number of neurological symptoms. By suspending the Lyme-trained doctor's medical license, the Swedish government has created obstacles to care for this child and all those suffering from this infection.

Colonel Nicole Malachowski had nearly two decades of experience as an officer, leader, and fighter pilot in the United States Air Force when she was infected with Lyme borreliosis. She is among the first group of women to fly modern military fighter planes and led a fighter squadron. The Colonel testified before US federal officials in December 2017 as to how this infection nearly broke her. As her symptoms increased in range, frequency and intensity, this intelligent woman, of proven competence and bravery under life-and-death situations, was told she 'could not handle stress' by professionals in the military and private healthcare systems. The Colonel's debilitating symptoms were dismissed, and her person was discredited and trivialized. It was 'by luck' that she found medical professionals that were competent to diagnose and treat her with protocols that included many months of antimicrobials … despite the risk of being harassed or punished for going against the previous physicians' assumptions and for ultimately fulfilling the Hippocratic oath.

Research in Africa found pathogenic borreliosis infections are widespread across the continent and West African patients who had been misdiagnosed with drug resistant malaria subsequently showed undiagnosed borreliosis infection. The medical infrastructure in Africa is less robust than that of Europe and the US. However, patients with financial resources sufficient to seek and secure their diagnosis can usually access antimicrobial treatments that are appropriate to their symptoms. As with other stubborn bacterial infections, they can pay for treatment

i

© Copyright 2018. Global Network on Institutional Discrimination and
Ad Hoc Committee for Health Equity in ICD11 Borreliosis Codes. All Rights Reserved

until their symptoms are greatly reduced or gone. The numbers of persons in Africa with pathogenic borreliosis infection who have the resources to secure diagnosis and treatment remains unknown.

The numbers of persons with Lyme and relapsing fever borreliosis who are able to secure diagnosis and treatment also remains unknown in the US. Late Texas Senator Chris Harris suffered for many years from a range of 'unexplained symptoms' after his 1990 Lyme diagnosis. The Senator was then diagnosed with late stage systemic Lyme. During this time, the Texas state medical authorities, and medical authorities across the US, were attacking doctors that did not follow the restrictive Infectious Diseases Society of America (IDSA) clinical guidelines for Lyme. They were suspending doctors' licenses and penalizing them for spurious complaints such as unspecified or fallacious record-keeping concerns, and were penalizing them with substantial fines and time-consuming, intrusive and arbitrary tasks. Almost all of these actions were initiated by private health insurance complaints that used IDSA doctors as expert witnesses to deny coverage for non-IDSA protocols. The Senator's doctor arranged for 17 physicians to take turns writing one-month prescriptions for antibiotics to treat this systemic infection. In an interview before his death, the Senator acknowledged Lyme disease 'rotted out his bones and gave him a heart attack.' He said, "As a Lyme disease survivor, I know how important the correct treatment can be." The Senator was clearly not referring to the IDSA treatment guidelines when he made this statement.

The four examples provided demonstrate some of the context regarding how human rights violations are experienced by the human rights defenders of Lyme and relapsing fever borreliosis patients.

This report will show how conflicts of interest, market competition, State Actor collusion with private sector profiteers and other nonmedical and non-science-based dynamics are destroying the capacity to provide care for estimated millions living with Lyme and relapsing fever borreliosis infections.

The results are many medical practitioners and scientists devoted to under-standing this illness and treating these patients are routinely defamed, their freedoms to associate and speak restricted, and they are threatened with the loss of their livelihoods.

Most people recognize the devotion to human rights of the journalist who goes into a war zone to find and share the truth of innocent people brutalized by war crimes and by the persons who organize to free children from international sex

© Copyright 2018. Global Network on Institutional Discrimination and
Ad Hoc Committee for Health Equity in ICD11 Borreliosis Codes. All Rights Reserved

trafficking. These defenders of human rights can be easily identified because they are working to address situations we all can recognize as horrific.

In contrast, the healthcare systems across the globe are largely recognized as flawed but not intentionally horrendous. However, increasing numbers of scholarly publications have documented how these healthcare systems have become quietly corrupted and call these comfortable beliefs into question.

There is universal agreement that prisoners have a right to medical care. Precisely what is the difference between a 'prisoner of war' and 'an eight-year-old boy' being denied medically necessary antimicrobial care?

Seizing the business of a political opposition party leader is prohibited. Precisely what is the difference between 'seizing the businesses from a political opposition party leader' and a medical board with members representing one medical society 'closing down the business of a medical doctor that belongs to a competing medical society'?

Precisely what is the difference between a crime of 'physical assault by policemen against innocent citizens' and corrupted governmental policies that assault patient rights' to informed consent, diagnosis and treatment options? Both are acts of brutality by State Actors that result in unnecessary physical harm and suffering.

Every time a human rights defender for Lyme and relapsing fever borreliosis patients is attacked and removed, an estimated 10,000 or more borreliosis patients will lose access to proper diagnosis and medical care that meets internationally accepted standards.

Jenna Luché-Thayer
Founder and Director,
Ad Hoc Committee for Health Equity in ICD11 Borreliosis Codes

iii

© Copyright 2018. Global Network on Institutional Discrimination and
Ad Hoc Committee for Health Equity in ICD11 Borreliosis Codes. All Rights Reserved

SUMMARY

On October 24, 2017, the United Nations (UN) Special Rapporteur (SR) on the right to health, Dainius Pūras, presented his report on corruption to the UN General Assembly. He told his audience, "In many countries, health is among the most corrupt sectors; this has significant implications for equality and non-discrimination "... He noted some are related to the global pharmaceutical industry and others from "institutional corruption" and emphasized the "normalization" of corruption in healthcare which includes practices undermining medical ethics, social justice, transparency and effective healthcare provision, as well as illegal acts. Many researchers and scholars support the SR's findings and note how the corporatization of medical practice has contributed to this situation and the loss of medical professional autonomy.

Many governments now recognize that healthcare and disability costs are unsustainable and may undermine their national economies. Nevertheless, current practices regarding healthcare cost considerations are largely reduced to insurers' quarterly earnings and governments' annual budgets.

This short-term thinking is disastrous with regards to the unsustainable healthcare and disability costs from the expanding pandemic of undiagnosed, misdiagnosed, untreated and/or undertreated Lyme and relapsing fever borreliosis patients.

Affordable access to all treatment options that meet international standards and a variety of diagnostic tests will greatly reduce this projected burden. Further-more, properly recognizing and addressing the Lyme and relapsing fever borreliosis pandemic will serve economic and humanitarian goals.

Borreliosis is a disease caused by infection by bacteria named *Borrelia*. All known forms of borreliosis are zoonotic and transmitted to humans through exposure to vector organisms. The World Health Organization (WHO) has recognized Lyme borreliosis as a multi-region 'disease of consequence' for decades. Nevertheless, across the globe, State response to one of the most prevalent and rapidly spreading infectious diseases of our time is the cause of unnecessary suffering.

This poor healthcare response is not happening because better methods of diagnosis and treatment do not exist —in fact they do. It is happening because

© Copyright 2018. Global Network on Institutional Discrimination and
Ad Hoc Committee for Health Equity in ICD11 Borreliosis Codes. All Rights Reserved

of corruption, conflicts of interest and unethical practices that are ignored or even promoted by State Actors, their agents and vested business interests.

Clinicians and researchers across the US, Canada, Eastern, Western and Northern Europe, the Asia Pacific and Africa have stated that WHO's international diagnostic codes (ICD) for Lyme and relapsing fever borrelioses need to be updated and expanded to better reflect the state of the science regarding these diseases. These limited and outdated codes result in very sick people being denied treatment —even when treatment options come from clinical practice guidelines that meet internationally accepted standards for guidelines, such as the 2011 standards set by Institute of Medicine (IOM or US National Academies of Sciences, Engineering and Medicine). Until this happens, estimated millions of people will suffer needlessly.

This under-addressed pandemic is generating a host of unsustainable conditions that are undermining economic development, human dignity and human rights. Furthermore, there are many indications that these diseases will exacerbate with climate change.

The Ad Hoc Committee for Health Equity in ICD11 Borreliosis Codes was formed in 2016 to update WHO's ICD codes for Lyme borreliosis and to demonstrate how the outdated and restrictive codes have been contributing to human rights violations. Their principal report, Updating ICD11 Borreliosis Diagnostic Codes, was accepted by WHO and was also submitted to Dainius Pūras, the UN Human Rights Council's Special Rapporteur (SR) for the right of everyone to the enjoyment of the highest attainable standard of physical and mental health.

The Ad Hoc Committee met with the SR in his official capacity on June 7, 2017. The SR heard the Committee's testimony as to how medical practitioners had collectively and effectively treated tens of thousands of patients with persistent and complicated LB and documentation including that which shows the many potential complications of borrelial infections.

These materials firmly establish the significant possibility that patients with persistent LB require biological medical care —not as a matter of opinion, but as a matter of scientific fact. The record also shows many different types of health human rights violations. These include obstruction of access to treatment options from clinical practice guidelines that meet internationally accepted standards for guidelines. The WHO diagnostic codes for LB are a significant driver of these human rights violations. The codes are outdated, of limited scope and detail, are inappropriately restrictive and:

v

© Copyright 2018. Global Network on Institutional Discrimination and
Ad Hoc Committee for Health Equity in ICD11 Borreliosis Codes. All Rights Reserved

- prevent proper diagnosis and obstruct access to treatment options that meet internationally accepted standards,
  - ➢ e.g. deny LB screening requests made by pregnant women and deny treatment options to pregnant women who have LB infections; infections proven to be cross the placenta and cause severe negative outcomes to babies including miscarriage, stillbirth and sudden infant death syndrome (SIDS)
- promote discrimination based on illness manifestations that are not included in current codes
- restrict information regarding the availability of treatment options that meet internationally accepted standards
- obstruct treatments directed toward illness manifestations that are not included in current codes
- promote discrimination based on financial status
- support attacks on human rights defenders —including medical practitioners, scientists and researchers who act on behalf of this vulnerable patient group
- routinely exclude key stakeholders —such as medical practitioners, researchers, patients and caretakers who are concerned with persistent and complicated cases of LB —from decision-making venues … making these stakeholders invisible to policy makers, economists and other practitioners and researchers
- misapply 'psychosomatic disorder' diagnoses and deny care for biological illness in lieu of medical diagnosis and care for biological illness[1]
- sick children receiving treatments that meet internationally accepted standards are forcibly removed from their parents who are falsely accused of criminal acts, such as poisoning their children, or Münchhausen by proxy syndrome (a highly disputed diagnosis that indicates gender bias)
- alarming cases where euthanasia is encouraged over therapies that meet internationally accepted standards

Congenital Lyme disease, persistent infection, borrelial lymphocytoma, granuloma annulare, morphea, localized scleroderma, lichen sclerosis and atrophicus, Lyme meningitis, Lyme nephritis, Lyme hepatitis, Lyme myositis, Lyme aortic aneurysm, coronary artery aneurysm, late Lyme endocarditis, Lyme carditis, late Lyme neuritis or neuropathy, meningo-vascular borreliosis and neuroborreliosis – with cerebral infarcts, intracranial aneurysm, Lyme Parkinsonism, late Lyme meningoen-cephalitis or meningo-myeloencephalitis, atrophic form of Lyme meningoen-cephalitis with dementia and subacute presenile dementia, neuro-psychiatric manifestations, late Lyme disease of liver and other viscera, late Lyme disease of kidney and ureter, late Lyme disease of bronchus and lung and seronegative and latent Lyme disease, unspecified.

---

[1] These psychosomatic disorder concepts have been repudiated by the American Psychiatric Association or APA.

© Copyright 2018. Global Network on Institutional Discrimination and Ad Hoc Committee for Health Equity in ICD11 Borreliosis Codes. All Rights Reserved

<u>The Situation of Human Rights Defenders of Lyme and Relapsing Fever Borreliosis Patients: Edition One</u> was developed as a complementary report to <u>Updating ICD11 Borreliosis Diagnostic Codes: Edition One</u>.

This 'borreliosis patients' defenders report' details some of the complex global relationships and financial incentives driving additional human rights violations of those who defend this patient community. It was written for submission to SR Dainius Pūras and SR Michel Forst, the SR responsible for the "Declaration on the Right and Responsibility of Individuals, Groups and Organs of Society to Promote and Protect Universally Recognized Human Rights and Fundamental Freedoms" or the 'situation of human rights defenders'.

The report includes detailed case studies from many countries as to how these rights are being violated and highlights how:
- scientific and medical knowledge has been ignored and/or suppressed through the actions of State Actors, intergovernmental bodies and certain medical societies; inaccurate and misleading scientific and medical messages have been promoted and allowed to proliferate
- The defenders —including medical practitioners, scientists, laboratory owners and the parents of children with these illnesses— routinely experience aggressive opposition and attacks by State Actors, State-sponsored entities and affiliated business interests
- The costs of Lyme Borreliosis are underestimated. For example, 36 percent of those infected will develop long-term illness that is often not covered by insurance or national health systems. Another example: the many people with LB who have been wrongly diagnosed with incurable conditions such as multiple sclerosis, lupus and dementia and therefore wrongfully treated with expensive, potentially dangerous and in these cases ineffective disease modifying drugs
- The global role of the Infectious Diseases Society of America (IDSA) as a powerful business interest is noted, e.g. how it implements an international strategy to maintain their LB opinions and assists:
  - insurers and State Actors in off-loading care costs onto patients
  - their European colleagues in maintaining market dominance through bodies such as: European Union Concerted Action on Lyme Borreliosis (EUCALB), and European Society of Clinical Microbiology and Infectious Diseases' (ESCMID) Study Group for Lyme Borreliosis (ESGBOR).
  - State Actors and other medical societies to base their Lyme guidelines on the 2006 IDSA Lyme Guidelines that are elaborated as a case study in conflicts of interest, medical and scientific bias and other poor practices in the IOM's 2011 <u>Clinical Practice Guidelines We Can Trust</u> (page 56, BOX 3-1)

© Copyright 2018. Global Network on Institutional Discrimination and
Ad Hoc Committee for Health Equity in ICD11 Borreliosis Codes. All Rights Reserved

- routinely makes false accusations against its competitors, e.g. falsely accuses competitors of making death threats in a PowerPoint presentation at an international conference
- in the suppression of science —for example, IDSA and their associates acknowledge a complex LB illness in their patent applications, however, they openly deny or minimize this information in published materials and public opinions— the language in many of these patents directly oppose the claims and opinions making up the 2006 guidelines.

The situation of Lyme and relapsing fever borreliosis patients and their defenders show violations in eleven human rights treatises and articles pertaining to the rights to: freedom from torture and cruel, inhuman and degrading treatment; freedom of association; participation in public policy; due process and remedy; liberty and security of person; privacy and confidentiality; bodily integrity; the highest attainable standard of health; nondiscrimination and equality; and parents defending their rights to prohibit the administration of medicine to a child against parents' wishes.

© Copyright 2018. Global Network on Institutional Discrimination and
Ad Hoc Committee for Health Equity in ICD11 Borreliosis Codes. All Rights Reserved

TABLE OF CONTENTS

© Copyright 2018. Global Network on Institutional Discrimination and
Ad Hoc Committee for Health Equity in ICD11 Borreliosis Codes. All Rights Reserved

© Copyright 2018. Global Network on Institutional Discrimination and
Ad Hoc Committee for Health Equity in ICD11 Borreliosis Codes. All Rights Reserved

I.   Introduction

"recognition of the inherent dignity and of the equal and inalienable rights of all members of the human family is the foundation of freedom, justice and peace in the world"
—stated principle in the
1948 Universal Declaration of Human Rights

Across the globe, State response to one of the most prevalent and rapidly spreading infectious diseases of our time is the cause of unnecessary suffering. This suffering is caused by the lack of diagnosis and misdiagnoses. Unless they have the resources to pay for private specialist care, those who receive a proper diagnosis are denied treatment options that have met stringent internationally accepted standards, and are limited to protocols that are arbitrary, restrictive and often not curative ...with the result being ongoing illness, progressive debility, disability and death.

This poor healthcare response is not happening because better methods of diagnosis and treatment do not exist —in fact they do. It is happening because of corruption, conflicts of interest and unethical practices that are ignored or even promoted by State Actors, their agents and business interests. As a result, the basic human rights of literally millions of people are being violated.

Borreliosis is a disease caused by infection by bacteria named *Borrelia*. Borrelioses are considered to belong to one of two groups, relapsing fever and Lyme borreliosis, which have a worldwide distribution and may be considered pandemic. The World Health Organization (WHO) has recognized Lyme borreliosis as a multi-region 'disease of consequence' for decades.

In August 2017, the European Centre for Disease Prevention and Control (ECDC) published a report stating that Lyme borreliosis (LB) is among the 30 most threatening diseases for public health. According to the

October 24, 2017, The United Nations (UN) Special Rapporteur (SR) on the right to health, Dainius Pūras presented his report on corruption to the UN General Assembly.

He told his audience, "In many countries, health is among the most corrupt sectors, this has significant implications for equality and non-discrimination ..."

He noted domestic and global root causes of corruption, including those related to the pharmaceutical industry, others from "institutional corruption".

He emphasized the "normalization" of corruption in healthcare which includes practices undermining medical ethics, social justice, transparency and effective healthcare provision, as well as illegal acts. [1]

© Copyright 2018. Global Network on Institutional Discrimination and
Ad Hoc Committee for Health Equity in ICD11 Borreliosis Codes. All Rights Reserved

European Union (Decision 1082/2013/EU), LB is a "serious cross-border threat to health … [and] may necessitate coordination at Union level in order to ensure a high level of human health protection".

All known forms of borreliosis are zoonotic and transmitted to humans through exposure to vector organisms. For LB, there are also cases of interhuman transmission such as congenital transmission [2] [3] [4] [5] [6] [7] [8].

Experts across key veterinary and medical institutions in West Africa have stated that many communities across the continent of Africa depend on livestock for their livelihood and thus are at high risk of borreliosis. Furthermore, research has shown that many cases of what was assumed to be drug resistant malaria were in fact illnesses that could be attributed to borreliosis.

Medical and scientific professionals have noted that thousands of Australian patients show symptoms of tick-borne diseases including those caused by *Borrelia species pluralis* or spp. Existing diagnostic tests are limited in their ability to identify persons with borreliosis caused by species such as these which differ slightly from that which causes Lyme disease. The resultant lack of diagnostic tools for variant forms of *Borrelia* that may cause 'Lyme-like' illness leave many Australian patients without a diagnosis and therefore without access to medical care.

Clinicians and researchers across the North and South America, Eastern, Western and Northern Europe, the Asia Pacific and Africa have stated that WHO's international diagnostic codes (ICD) for Lyme and relapsing fever borrelioses need to be updated and expanded to better reflect the state of the science regarding these diseases.

Across the globe, medical systems use the WHO diagnostic codes to categorize illness and determine treatments. These limited and outdated borreliosis codes result in very sick people being denied treatment —even when treatment options come from clinical practice guidelines that meet internationally accepted standards for guidelines, such as the 2011 standards set by Institute of Medicine (IOM or US National Academies of Sciences, Engineering and Medicine). Furthermore, the WHO diagnostic codes do not recognize many of the disabling conditions caused by these infections [9][10].

According to West African and Australian medical and scientific professionals, the current codes for relapsing fever and Lyme-like illness are misinforming those trying to help these patients —this results in inadequate, wrongful or no medical care. For example, the ICD-10 definition of Relapsing Fever Borreliosis excludes critical information such as:

2

© Copyright 2018. Global Network on Institutional Discrimination and
Ad Hoc Committee for Health Equity in ICD11 Borreliosis Codes. All Rights Reserved

✓ new geno-species of relapsing fever *Borrelia*, e.g. *B. miyamotoi* which has been found to vector both soft and hard ticks

✓ relapsing fever borreliosis and Lyme Borreliosis have stages of dissemination and multiple varieties of symptoms afflicting multiple bodily systems in relapsing remitting fashion —similar to syphilis, another spirochetal infection

Updating the WHO's codes used by medical professionals will additionally improve disease surveillance. Until this happens, estimated millions of people will suffer needlessly [10].

There has been inadequate response by key State Actors and intergovernmental bodies to the epidemic of Lyme and relapsing fever borrelioses. For example, certain European governments have set arbitrary ceilings for the number of LB cases that may be reported in any given time period and others make little effort to collect this surveillance data. Such practices have contributed to inaccurate and artificially low LB surveillance numbers. These unreliable numbers then contribute to a misinformed and inadequate government response to the disease.

The inadequate response by State Actors and intergovernmental bodies to this human suffering has had consequences. One result is organizing by civil society to address this pandemic and hold governments and intergovernmental bodies accountable. These consequences will be further detailed in this report.

Apart from the medical and scientific professionals who are concerned with providing diagnosis and therapies for this patient group, this civil society movement has increasing numbers of individuals with extensive scientific, medical, or professional experience who are also assessing the political and economic influences interfering with implementing a practical and humane response to the pandemic.

In addition, there are increasing numbers of individuals and organizations that are implementing concrete legal and political action to correct the inadequate response by intergovernmental bodies and State Actors.

> *"A very large proportion of the activities of human rights defenders can be characterized as acting in support of victims of human rights violations"* …
> —UN Office of the High Commissioner for Human Rights (OHCR) [11]

Among those involved in these peaceful actions are the human rights defenders of those living with Lyme and/or relapsing fever borreliosis. The defenders — including medical practitioners, scientists, laboratory owners and the parents of children with these illnesses— routinely experience aggressive opposition by State

3

© Copyright 2018. Global Network on Institutional Discrimination and
Ad Hoc Committee for Health Equity in ICD11 Borreliosis Codes. All Rights Reserved

Actors, State-sponsored entities and affiliated business interests that qualify as human rights violations.

This under-addressed pandemic is generating a host of unsustainable conditions that are undermining economic development, human dignity and human rights. Furthermore, there are many indications that these diseases will exacerbate with climate change [12] [13] [14] [15] [16] [17] [18] [19] [20] [21] [22].

It was these concerns that prompted action on the part of the Ad Hoc Committee for Health Equity in ICD11 Borreliosis Codes (or Ad Hoc Committee). The Ad Hoc Committee is part of the global borreliosis community and includes nongovernmental organizations, scientists, medical professionals, patient groups, government officials and elected officials [23].

The Ad Hoc Committee was formed in 2016 to update WHO's ICD codes for Lyme borreliosis and to demonstrate how the outdated and restrictive codes have been contributing to human rights violations.

The Ad Hoc Committee is concerned with bacterial infections that lead to human illness, such as Lyme borreliosis or Lyme disease which are caused by multiple species of spirochetes from the *Borrelia burgdorferi sensu lato* complex and relapsing fever *Borrelia* species, both of which are distributed worldwide. They are also concerned with tick-borne disease co-infections including *Babesia, Bartonella, Anaplasma,* and *Ehrlichia* as well as opportunistic viral, parasitic and fungal infections.

The members of the Ad Hoc Committee are human rights defenders. Their principal report, Updating ICD11 Borreliosis Diagnostic Codes, was accepted by WHO and was also submitted to Dainius Pūras, the UN Human Rights Council's Special Rapporteur (SR) for the right of everyone to the enjoyment of the highest attainable standard of physical and mental health [10].

The Ad Hoc Committee met with the SR in his official capacity on June 7, 2017. The SR accepted all the Committee's documentation including reports, books and videos, PowerPoint and verbal testimony; his Senior Human Rights Officer and Team Leader put them into record. Dainius Pūras also told the Ad Hoc Committee how he could support their efforts within the framework of his mandate.

The record now includes hundreds of peer-reviewed studies —written by nationally and internationally recognized scientists and medical researchers from across the globe— that describe the many potential complications of borrelial infections:

© Copyright 2018. Global Network on Institutional Discrimination and
Ad Hoc Committee for Health Equity in ICD11 Borreliosis Codes. All Rights Reserved

Congenital Lyme disease, persistent infection, borrelial lymphocytoma, granuloma annulare, morphea, localized scleroderma, lichen sclerosis and atrophicus, Lyme meningitis, Lyme nephritis, Lyme hepatitis, Lyme myositis, Lyme aortic aneurysm, coronary artery aneurysm, late Lyme endocarditis, Lyme carditis, late Lyme neuritis or neuropathy, meningovascular borreliosis and neuroborreliosis – with cerebral infarcts, intracranial aneurysm, Lyme Parkinsonism, late Lyme meningoencephalitis or meningomyelo-encephalitis, atrophic form of Lyme meningoencephalitis with dementia and subacute presenile dementia, neuropsychiatric manifestations, late Lyme disease of liver and other viscera, late Lyme disease of kidney and ureter, late Lyme disease of bronchus and lung and seronegative and latent Lyme disease, unspecified [2].

The Committee members then gave verbal and additional written testimony as to how medical practitioners on the Committee had <u>collectively and effectively treated tens of thousands of patients with persistent and complicated LB with clinical practice guidelines that meet internationally accepted standards</u>.

These materials firmly establish the significant possibility that patients with persistent LB require biological medical care —not as a matter of opinion, but as a matter of scientific fact.

Furthermore, therapies for persistent Lyme —including extended and combination antimicrobial therapies that have met internationally recognized standards for clinical guidelines— are available, as are accredited educational programs on how to implement such therapies, extensive training programs for healthcare professionals, and other resources.

The record also shows many different types of health human rights violations. These include obstruction of access to treatment options from clinical practice guidelines that meet internationally accepted standards for guidelines.

This obstruction to access violates the Availability, Accessibility, Acceptability, Quality (AAAQ) of Health Human Rights imperatives for "non-discriminatory" practices and medical ethics. The principle of Affordability is found under Accessibility. Currently, access to treatment options that meet internationally accepted standards is limited to those who can afford to pay with private funds as most health insurers and national health services have policies to refuse this coverage.

---

[2] No medical condition was entered into the report if it had less than three supporting peer-reviewed publications.

© Copyright 2018. Global Network on Institutional Discrimination and
Ad Hoc Committee for Health Equity in ICD11 Borreliosis Codes. All Rights Reserved

Lyme borreliosis (LB) is a clinical diagnosis, meaning the patient's history and clinical presentation can be diagnostic, and laboratory tests are not required but may be supportive. Despite this, the record shows how LB patients who have received an appropriate clinical diagnosis are routinely denied care should unreliable laboratory tests fail to confirm their clinical diagnosis.

The WHO diagnostic codes for LB are a significant driver of these human rights violations. The codes are outdated, of limited scope and detail, and are inappropriately restrictive. These codes are linked to policies recommending practices that, for many patients:

- prevent proper diagnosis and obstruct access to treatment options that meet internationally accepted standards,
  - e.g. deny LB screening requests made by pregnant women and deny treatment options to pregnant women who have LB infections; infections proven to be cross the placenta and cause severe negative outcomes to babies including miscarriage, stillbirth and sudden infant death syndrome (SIDS) [24]

- promote discrimination based on illness manifestations that are not included in current codes

> ### PART I. Abuse of Psychosomatic Diagnosis
>
> Following his June 2017 report to the UN Human Rights Council in Geneva, SR Dainius Pūras noted that mental health policies and services are in crisis of power imbalances.
>
> He said there was a "grossly unmet" need for rights-based care and support and that huge power imbalances in the systems, supported by the pharmaceutical industry, perpetuate the "biased" use of evidence and excessive use of psychotropic medicines, that people experiencing mental distress and diagnosed with "mental disorders" are dangerous.
>
> According to Dainius Pūras, "These concepts perpetuate stigma and discrimination, as well as the practices of coercion." [25]

- restrict information regarding the availability of treatment options that meet internationally accepted standards

- obstruct treatments based on illness manifestations that are not included in current codes

- promote discrimination based on financial status

- support attacks on human rights defenders —including medical practitioners, scientists and researchers who act on behalf of this vulnerable patient group

6

© Copyright 2018. Global Network on Institutional Discrimination and
Ad Hoc Committee for Health Equity in ICD11 Borreliosis Codes. All Rights Reserved

- routinely exclude key stakeholders —such as medical practitioners, researchers, patients and caretakers who are concerned with persistent and complicated cases of LB —from decision-making venues … making these stakeholders invisible to policy makers, economists and other practitioners and researchers

- misapply 'psychosomatic disorder' diagnoses and deny care for biological illness in lieu of medical diagnosis and care for biological illness [3] [26]

- sick children receiving treatments that meet internationally accepted standards are forcibly removed from their parents who are falsely accused of criminal acts, such as poisoning their children, or Münchhausen by proxy syndrome (a highly disputed diagnosis that indicates gender bias) [27]

- alarming cases where euthanasia is encouraged over therapies that meet internationally accepted standards

> **PART II. Abuse of Psychosomatic Diagnosis**
>
> Thousands of documented cases on record with multiple governments report how the obstruction to diagnosis and treatments cause LB patients and those suffering from Lyme-like illness severe psychosocial and financial distress.
>
> This suffering is often responded to by practices and policies that are corrupted, e.g. such patients are mislabeled with having psychosomatic conditions rather than biological illness.
>
> These mislabeled patients are often forced to take psychotropic medicines.

The human rights defenders of this patient group are routinely threatened and punished. This includes medical professionals who are fulfilling their Hippocratic oath to this marginalized patient community. This threat awareness results in many medical professionals and scientists avoiding or rejecting this patient group.

Despite these threats and personal jeopardy, the defenders have assisted tens of thousands of patients with persistent and complicated Lyme and relapsing fever borreliosis to regain their quality of life, manage their illness and become productive and contributing members of society.

The widespread discrimination experienced by Lyme and relapsing fever patients has been systemic and institutionalized across ICD codes, national health policies and medical and insurance systems. Altogether, these factors have led to gross human rights violations that are on record with the UN Human Rights Council's SR for the right of everyone to the enjoyment of the highest attainable standard of physical and mental health.

---

[3] These psychosomatic disorder concepts have been repudiated by the American Psychiatric Association or APA.

© Copyright 2018. Global Network on Institutional Discrimination and
Ad Hoc Committee for Health Equity in ICD11 Borreliosis Codes. All Rights Reserved

However, the Ad Hoc Committee recognizes that the complex global tentacles of these violations require additional documentation as well as additional recognition and support from the United Nations Office of the High Commissioner for Human Rights.

As a result, the Ad Hoc Committee determined it was essential for both SR Dainius Pūras and SR Michel Forst, the SR responsible for the "Declaration on the Right and Responsibility of Individuals, Groups and Organs of Society to Promote and Protect Universally Recognized Human Rights and Fundamental Freedoms" or the 'situation of human rights defenders', be apprised of the situation of those defending the health human rights of this patient group.

Therefore, The Situation of Human Rights Defenders of Lyme and Relapsing Fever Borreliosis Patients: Edition One was developed as a complementary report to Updating ICD11 Borreliosis Diagnostic Codes: Edition One.

II.   Overview of the Situation

There are more than four decades of practices, by many different institutions, that have shaped the response to the pandemic of Lyme and relapsing fever borrelioses, and the current situation of its human rights defenders and their patients.

One result is that Lyme borreliosis is the only known infectious disease whereby licensed practitioners, treating patients according to guidelines that meet internationally accepted standards, are constantly at risk for defamation and restrictions made to their movement, speech and associational life, unfair due process, restrictions on their medical practices, and the loss of their licenses and livelihoods.

Corruption and Fraud

In this report, the terms corruption and fraud are based upon the concepts and practices elaborated in the following documents and related policies and treatises:

> In his presentation to the UN General Assembly on October 22, 2015, Michel Forst, SR for the 'situation of defenders' spoke of the global trends affecting human rights defenders.
>
> Michel Forst was struck by the 'interconnectedness of the multiple threats encountered by defenders' as well as the increase in attacks on individual defenders, the implementation of new intimidation and repressive measures, especially the use of laws to circumscribe and delegitimize the work of defenders ... and ... the "numerous institutional weaknesses of certain States." [28]

© Copyright 2018. Global Network on Institutional Discrimination and
Ad Hoc Committee for Health Equity in ICD11 Borreliosis Codes. All Rights Reserved

- 2004 United Nations Convention against Corruption which followed the October 31, 2003 General Assembly resolution 58/4 to develop and support a comprehensive United Nations Convention against Corruption [29]
- September 1, 2016 Anti-Fraud and Anti-Corruption Framework for the United Nations Secretariat [30]

The concepts include expectations for all members of society including:

- codes of conduct for public officials
- requirements for transparent and accountable public reporting by State Actors private sector regulations and participation of society
- fraudulent acts and conflicts of interests
- distinguishes illegal trading in influence wherein 'improper influence' shows 'corrupt intent' from legal lobbying
- 'preventing the misuse of procedures regulating private entities, including procedures regarding subsidies and licenses granted by public authorities for commercial activities'
- 'promoting the development of standards and procedures designed to safeguard the integrity of relevant private entities, including codes of conduct for the correct, honorable and proper performance of the activities of business and all relevant professions and the prevention of conflicts of interest, and for the promotion of the use of good commercial practices among businesses and in the contractual relations of businesses with the State'
- and so forth

Practices that create corruption vary. The global organization Transparency International (Denmark) defines corruption as "misuse of trusted authority for own sake". Transparency International finds "corruption is a problem because it ... dilutes confidence in democracy's main institutions and violates fundamental equality principles. Transparency International notes that "studies show that there is a close correlation between the perceived corruption and the actual corruption."

II.1. Policies, Treatises and Laws that Pertain

There are numerous UN Treatises as well as UN and member State policies and laws that pertain to the situation of the defenders and those patients they defend. A key example is the UN's Sustainable Development Goals (SDG) 2015-2030 which include Goal #3 "to ensure healthy lives and promote well-being for all at all ages". The SDG supports the Right to Health as a fundamental right enshrined

© Copyright 2018. Global Network on Institutional Discrimination and
Ad Hoc Committee for Health Equity in ICD11 Borreliosis Codes. All Rights Reserved

within the international human rights framework of the imperative of Availability, Accessibility, Acceptability, Quality (AAAQ) of care [31] [32] [33].

In his 2016 annual report to the UN General Assembly, Dainius Pūras, the SR on the right to health, noted synergies between improving the right to health and attaining SDGs [34]. The SR noted that almost all the SDG's Goals can be linked to health, underlined the necessity of a well-functioning health system, and noted that States are legally obligated to "devote maximum available resources to the right to health".

The SR presented key challenges that affect developed and developing countries alike; these issues include inequity and equality. He stated, "The right to health requires States to prioritize vulnerable populations in terms of health resources, law and policy, participation and empowerment, and in disaggregated data."

On a global scale, the Lyme and relapsing fever patient group easily qualify as a vulnerable patient group. In the USA, Canada, Sweden, Denmark, Norway, Germany, France, the Netherlands, Belgium and many other nations, nearly every aspect of the right to health's AAAQ fails the LB patient group and undermines the situation of their human rights defenders.

"The right to health, like all human rights, imposes on the State Party three types of obligations [35]:

    Respect: This means simply not to interfere with the enjoyment of the right to health.
    Protect: This means ensuring that third parties (non-State Actors) do not infringe upon the enjoyment of the right to health.
    Fulfil: This means taking positive steps to realize the right to health."

"This must address the health concerns of the whole population; be devised, and periodically reviewed, on the basis of a participatory and transparent process; contain indicators and benchmarks by which progress can be closely monitored; and give particular attention to all vulnerable or marginalized groups ...

In this context, it is important to distinguish the *inability* from the *unwillingness* of a State Party to comply with its right to health obligations."

© Copyright 2018. Global Network on Institutional Discrimination and
Ad Hoc Committee for Health Equity in ICD11 Borreliosis Codes. All Rights Reserved

Chart: The Right to Health

"The right to health"

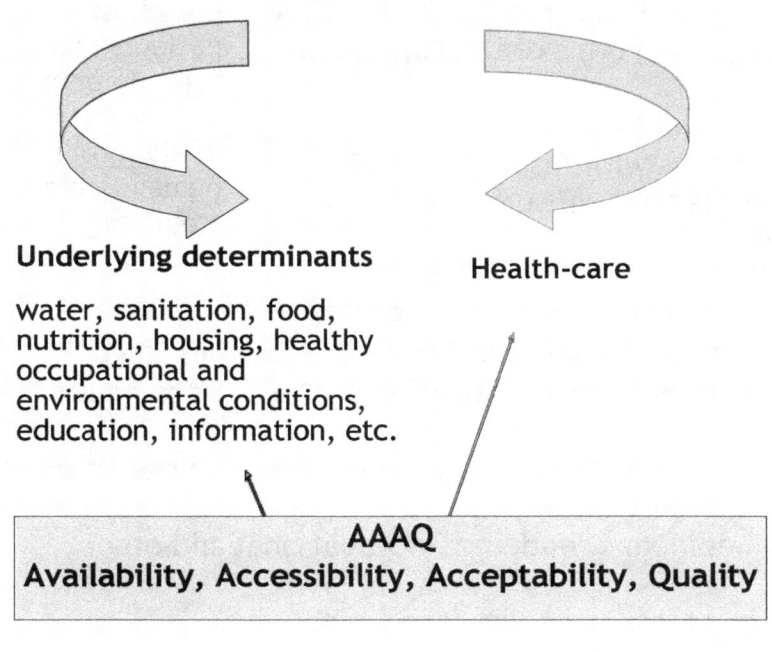

Underlying determinants

water, sanitation, food, nutrition, housing, healthy occupational and environmental conditions, education, information, etc.

Health-care

AAAQ
Availability, Accessibility, Acceptability, Quality

General Comment No. 14 of the Committee on Economic, Social and Cultural Rights

http://www.who.int/mediacentre/factsheets/fs323_en.pdf

Availability. Functioning public health and health care facilities, goods and services, as well as programs in sufficient quantity.

Accessibility. Health facilities, goods and services accessible to everyone within the jurisdiction of the State party.

Accessibility has four overlapping dimensions:

- non-discrimination
- physical accessibility
- economical accessibility or affordability
- information accessibility

Acceptability. All health facilities, goods and services must be respectful of medical ethics and culturally appropriate, as well as sensitive to gender and life-cycle requirements.

Quality Health facilities, goods and services must be scientifically and medically appropriate and of good quality.

II.1.1. Applicable Human Rights

Human dignity is the basis of fundamental human rights. Human dignity is inviolable and must be protected and respected. The dignity of the human person is a fundamental right in itself and constitutes the basis of fundamental rights in international law.

The human rights of LB patients and their human rights defenders are articulated in the many standards detailed in international and regional human rights norms and agreements. The pertinent human rights of Lyme and relapsing fever patients and their human rights defenders are found in the following international and regional treaties [36]:

11

© Copyright 2018. Global Network on Institutional Discrimination and
Ad Hoc Committee for Health Equity in ICD11 Borreliosis Codes. All Rights Reserved

- African Charter on Human and Peoples' Rights (ACHPR)
- Convention Against Torture (CAT)
- European Convention for the Prevention of Torture and Inhuman or Degrading Treatment or Punishment (ETS No.126)
- Convention on the Elimination of All Forms of Discrimination against Women (CEDAW)
- Convention on the Rights of the Child (CRC)
- Convention on the Rights of Persons with Disabilities (CRPD)
- European Convention on the Protection of Human Rights and Fundamental Freedoms (ECHR)
- European Social Charter (ESC)
- International Covenant on Civil and Political Rights (ICCPR)
- International Covenant on Economic, Social, and Cultural Rights (ICESCR) ICESCR's Article 12 states that steps for the realization of the right to health include those that:
  - ✓ reduce infant mortality and ensure the healthy development of the child;
  - ✓ improve environmental and industrial hygiene;
  - ✓ prevent, treat and control epidemic, endemic, occupational and other diseases;
  - ✓ create conditions to ensure access to health care for all.
- International Convention on the Elimination of All Forms of Racial Discrimination (ICERD)

> The situation of Lyme and relapsing fever borreliosis patients and their defenders show violations in **eleven** human rights treatises.

In addition, international standards now stipulate:

- ✓ The right to liberty and security of the person has been held to prohibit unauthorized disclosure of personal health data

- ✓ The rights to bodily integrity and security of the person have been held to prohibit the administration of medicine to a child against parents' wishes

- ✓ The right to freedom from cruel, inhuman, or degrading treatment or punishment has been held to oblige governments to secure the adequate health and well-being of prisoners

The following two tables, Table 1. Human Rights of Patients and Table 2. Human Rights of Human Right Defenders categorize the applicable human rights treaties and articles; article numbers are noted. The right to health includes the human rights in patient care as well as economic and political human rights that define the context of patient care provided by human rights defenders. Human rights defenders who are patients, as well as advocates, share all the rights noted in Table 1. Human Rights of Patients.

12

© Copyright 2018. Global Network on Institutional Discrimination and
Ad Hoc Committee for Health Equity in ICD11 Borreliosis Codes. All Rights Reserved

Table 1. Human Rights of Patients [37]

Human right	Treaty provisions	Examples of violations
Right to liberty and security of person	ICCPR 9(1), ACHPR 6, ECHR5(1)	LB patients are forced into psychiatric care for wrongful diagnosis of psychosomatic illness and denied medical care for persistent infection
Right to privacy and confidentiality	ICCPR 17(1), CRC 16(1), ECHR 8(1)	LB patient medical information is shared without their consent to State authorities who are harassing their doctors (human rights defenders) for providing LB patients treatment options that meet internationally accepted standards
Right to information	ICCPR 19(2), ACHPR 9, Council of Europe Framework Convention for the Protection of National Minorities (FCNM) 9(1), European Convention on Human Rights in Biomedicine (ECHRB) 5	<ul><li>The State fails to provide information regarding the risk of disability and death from undiagnosed and undertreated LB</li><li>The state routinely misinforms the public regarding the reliability of the diagnostic serology tests and increases their risk from disability and death from undiagnosed LB.</li><li>Practitioners fail to provide LB patients with information about treatment options and the potential risks and benefits of these options.</li></ul>
Right to bodily integrity[3]	ICERD 5(b), ACHPR 4, FCNM 6 (1), CRC 19(1), ECHRB 5	Practitioners fail to obtain free and informed consent from patients before treatments begin.
Right to life	ICCPR 6(1), ACHPR 4, ECHR 2(1)	<ul><li>Due to outdated and politicized State LB policies, disability, bankruptcy and suicide result for many LB patients.</li><li>Threats of loss of license and livelihood against doctors who treat LB patients according to protocols that have met internationally accepted standards results in many doctors turning away LB patients, leading to patient suicides and death.</li></ul>

---

[3] The right to bodily integrity is not specifically recognized under the ICCPR, ICESCR, ECHR, or ESC, but has been interpreted to be part of the right to security of the person, the right to freedom from torture and cruel, inhuman, and degrading treatment, and the right to the highest attainable standard of health.

13

© Copyright 2018. Global Network on Institutional Discrimination and
Ad Hoc Committee for Health Equity in ICD11 Borreliosis Codes. All Rights Reserved

Table 1. Human Rights of Patients (continued)

Human right	Treaty provisions	Examples of violations
Right to highest attainable standard of health	ICESCR 12, ICERD 5, CRC 24, CEDAW 12(1), ACHPR 16, ESC 11, ESC 13	▪ State health authorities allow insurers and state programs for low income families to deny medical care for persistent LB and LB complicated with co-infections. ▪ These policies result in obstruction to necessary medical care for those with insufficient economic resources to pay out-of-pocket for their medical care. ▪ Patients, who for financial reasons are limited to programs for low income families and coverage by insurance, are given inferior care.
Right to freedom from torture and cruel, inhuman and degrading treatment	ICCPR 7, CAT, ACHPR 5, ECHR 3, ETS No.126	State policies restricting antibiotic access for the bacterial infection caused by LB cause patients suffering from LB and co-infections to suffer unnecessary pain, disability, bankruptcy, and death.
Right to participation in public policy	ICCPR 25, ICERD 5(c) ACHPR 13(1), EFNM 15, CEDAW 7, CEDAW 14 (2)	▪ State funds and their partners disseminate articles that recommend LB patients and their human rights defenders be excluded from participating in LB-related policies. ▪ Participation in LB-related public policy by LB patients and their human rights defenders is 'empty theater' with no evidence of political commitment to change status quo and prioritize patient care, e.g. State colludes for wrongful financial incentives to drive preplanned outcome to suppress science and maintain status quo to deny breadth and seriousness of the epidemic, deny treatment based on clinical diagnosis and obstruct access to treatment options that meet internationally accepted standards.
Right to nondiscrimination and equality	ICCPR 21(1), ICCPR 26, ICESCR 2(2), ICERD, ACHPR 2 & 3, ACHPR 19, FCNM 4(1), ECHR 14, ECHRB 3	Medical practitioners, hospitals and policymakers are encouraged to claim LB patients have psychosomatic issues rather than biological illness and to obstruct access to medical care for infection and other complications.
Right to a remedy	ICCPR 2(3), ICERD 6, CEDAW 2, ACHPR 26, ECHR 13	The State takes no action to address any of the violations described above.

14

© Copyright 2018. Global Network on Institutional Discrimination and
Ad Hoc Committee for Health Equity in ICD11 Borreliosis Codes. All Rights Reserved

LB human rights defenders have the right to decent working conditions, the right to freedom of association and the right to liberty and security. Nevertheless, these defenders' economic and political human rights are routinely violated with both complicit and direct support from State Actors.

Table 2. Human Rights of Human Right Defenders [37]

Human right	Treaty provisions	Examples of violations
Right to freedom from torture and cruel, inhuman and degrading treatment	ICCPR 7, CAT, ACHPR 5, ECHR 3, ETS No.126	State Actors cause doctors mental and emotional anguish when they are forced to abandon their patients or barred from applying clinical practice guidelines that have been vetted through internationally accepted standards … this results in patients suffering from LB and co-infections to suffer unnecessary pain, disability, bankruptcy, and death.
Right to decent working conditions	ICESCR 7, ACHCR 15, ESC 2 through 4	Clinical practice guidelines of a professional medical society that have been vetted through internationally accepted standards and its members are defamed, harassed and threatened by members and State actors who belong to a competing medical society and their affiliates
Right to freedom of association	ICCPR 21, ACHPR 10, ECHR 5, 11	▪ Authorities use penalties to prevent practitioners who use guidelines that have been vetted through internationally accepted standards to travel to conferences ▪ Authorities prevent scientists from providing presentations who promote diagnostics tests that compete with the authorities (and their partners) patented tests
Right to participation in public policy	ICCPR 25, ICERD 5(c) ACHPR 13(1), EFNM 15, CEDAW 7, CEDAW 14 (2)	▪ State Actors fund and their partners disseminate articles that recommend LB patients and their human rights defenders be excluded from participating in LB-related policies. ▪ Participation in LB-related public policy by LB patients and their human rights defenders is 'empty theater' - collusion over wrongful financial incentives to drive preplanned policy outcomes to suppress science, harm patients and maintain status quo (see Table 1 for example)
Right rights to due process	ICCPR 14(1) ACHPR 7 ECHR 6(1)	▪ Practitioner facing disciplinary proceedings is unable to obtain access to all the evidence presented against him/her in advance of the hearing. ▪ A doctor in medical judgment suit has been put on strict limitations and not given a 'hearing' date two years after the commencement of the proceedings
Right to a remedy	ICCPR 2(3), ICERD 6, CEDAW 2, ACHPR 26, ECHR 13	The State takes no action to address any of the violations described above.

© Copyright 2018. Global Network on Institutional Discrimination and
Ad Hoc Committee for Health Equity in ICD11 Borreliosis Codes. All Rights Reserved

II.2. Scientific and Medical Knowledge has been Ignored or Suppressed

Through the actions of State Actors, intergovernmental bodies and certain medical societies, inaccurate and misleading scientific and medical messages have been allowed to proliferate, resulting in many literature reviews that recycle the same outdated and unsupported viewpoints and messages. These kinds of articles are published one or more times a year and are introduced onto many media platforms 'as new LB publications'.

On the other hand, the science and medical knowledge regarding persistent and complicated LB —derived from hundreds of peer reviewed publications written by nationally and internationally recognized experts— has been routinely ignored or suppressed by these State Actors, intergovernmental bodies, certain medical societies and editorial boards.

For example, LB is recognized as endemic in many areas of Europe and the USA, yet the science regarding the risk of contracting LB from blood transfusions is downplayed or ignored. According to the 2012 Blood donor selection: guidelines on assessing donor suitability for blood donation publication by WHO, "Endogenous bacteria that are transfusion-transmissible include *Treponema pallidum*, *Borrelia burgdorferi*, *Brucella melitensis* and *Yersinia enterocolitica*, but blood donations are routinely screened only for *T. pallidum* [syphilis]" [39].

> **Suppression of Science of Congenital Lyme**
>
> In the Sixth Edition of the Infectious Diseases of the Fetus and Newborn Infant, the 110-page chapter in Fifth Edition was removed and replaced with a 20-page chapter that basically negates congenital LB [38].
>
> Today, few obstetrics and gynecology professionals know congenital LB is a possibility.
>
> This is resulting in the death and disability of babies worldwide, from a treatable infection.

An example of this suppression is the denial of congenital LB infection as detailed in the medical reference textbooks Infectious Diseases of the Fetus and Newborn Infant, Fourth and Fifth Editions [40] [41].

In the Fifth Edition, a comprehensive chapter pertaining to the congenital transmission of LB was written by Dr. Tessa Gardner, a pediatric infectious disease (ID) specialist [5]. Gardner provided an extensive review of the significant body of

---

[5] Dr. Tessa Gardner, was a pediatric ID specialist in the Division of Pediatric Infectious Disease at St. John's Mercy Medical Centre and an Assistant Professor of Clinical Pediatrics with the Washington University School of Medicine in St. Louis, Missouri.

© Copyright 2018. Global Network on Institutional Discrimination and
Ad Hoc Committee for Health Equity in ICD11 Borreliosis Codes. All Rights Reserved

literature documenting the transplacental transmission of LB from pregnant mother to unborn child, with severe adverse outcomes including miscarriage and stillbirth. The 2001 Fifth Edition was over 110 pages long, with 888 scientific references. This knowledge is not present in the Sixth Edition.

Studies that show infections, including LB infections, may be a significant factor in complicated neurodegenerative diseases such as multiple sclerosis and Alzheimer's disease, and that their progression can be reversed or halted by extensive antimicrobial therapies. This information remains marginalized and is missing from government agencies, health systems and medical and scientific education.

Typically, these 'incurable' conditions are treated, often for life, with expensive and profitable disease modifying drugs. This is one reason why generic antimicrobial therapies, which have the potential to cure, are largely ignored by the many thousands of researchers, scientists and medical practitioners across the globe who receive grants and other benefits from Big Pharma [42] [43] [44].

Also ignored and suppressed are all the studies demonstrating the unreliability of the State Actors' recommended serology tests for LB [45] [46]. Studies have shown that these tests will miss two thirds of early cases (illness present for less than four weeks) and can miss up to half of late, established cases.

The responsible State Actors acknowledge that these serology tests are not very reliable at diagnosing early infection, yet at the same time, they require a positive test to confirm a diagnosis of Lyme borreliosis.

These practices by State Actors has resulted in not only missed diagnoses, but in hundreds of thousands of documented cases of treatment delay until the correct diagnosis was finally made. As a result, the infection was permitted to become fully systemic, making it far more difficult to effectively treat.

© Copyright 2018. Global Network on Institutional Discrimination and
Ad Hoc Committee for Health Equity in ICD11 Borreliosis Codes. All Rights Reserved

The CDC Acknowledged the Persistence and Complications of LB in 1991

In January 1991, the CDC published its official statement on LB. The 1991 CDC publication describes the complex, systemic, multi-symptom and sometimes devastating and chronic disease experienced by many LB patients, including those with co-infections [47].

The 1991 CDC publication recognizes:
- persistent LB infection and serious neurological complications
- the need to orient treatment to the individual case
- several antibiotics are effective and both oral and IV forms of antibiotics may be useful treatment.

The 1991 CDC publication states:
- "In some persons the rash never forms; in some, the first and only sign of Lyme disease is arthritis, and in others, nervous system problems are the only evidence of Lyme disease...
- Lyme disease is often difficult to diagnose because its symptoms and signs mimic those of many other diseases. Joint pain can be mistaken for other types of arthritis, such as rheumatoid arthritis, and neurologic signs can mimic those caused by other conditions, such as multiple sclerosis.
- Varying degrees of permanent damage to joints or the nervous system can develop in patients with late chronic Lyme disease. Typically, these are patients in whom Lyme disease was unrecognized in the early stages or for whom the initial treatment was unsuccessful.
- Antibiotics usually are given by mouth but may be given intravenously in more severe cases.
- In a few patients who are treated for Lyme disease, symptoms of persisting infection may continue or recur, making additional antibiotic treatment necessary.
- Rare deaths from Lyme disease have been reported.
- ...Lyme disease acquired during pregnancy may lead to infection of the fetus and possibly to stillbirth."

Key areas for research included:
- "Effects of mother's infection on the developing fetus.
- How Lyme disease bacteria cause chronic infections of the joints and nervous system and how to prevent these complications."

© Copyright 2018. Global Network on Institutional Discrimination and
Ad Hoc Committee for Health Equity in ICD11 Borreliosis Codes. All Rights Reserved

II.3. The Costs of Lyme Borreliosis are Underestimated

The suffering caused by Lyme and relapsing fever borreliosis has unknown overall cost— but studies indicate costs to be in the millions for employers and billions for certain national economies.

According to Swedish economist Marcus Davidson, the estimated treatment cost for Lyme disease for 2018 for Europe is between 10.1 billion and 20.1 billion euro (or 25.1 billion United States (US) dollars) and for the United States of America (USA) is between 4.8 billion and 9.6 billion US dollars [48].

This cost calculation does not include:

- the estimate that 36 percent of those infected will develop long-term illness [49] that is often not covered by insurance or national health systems

> One study estimates that chronic Lyme disease and associated diseases could be the cause of over 1200 suicides per year in the USA [50].

- the loss in productivity and increased liability and work-related accidents from compromised eyesight, hearing, cognition, judgement, strength, coordination and balance quite common to LB

- the many people with LB who have been wrongly diagnosed with incurable conditions such as multiple sclerosis, lupus and dementia and therefore wrongfully treated with expensive, potentially dangerous and in these cases ineffective disease modifying drugs

Furthermore, these cost calculations are also thwarted by the inaccuracy of the surveillance data. For example, the Dutch government report LB cases when the Erythema Migrans rash is observed whereas the Government of Ireland requires a serology confirmation from cerebral spinal fluid that shows neuroborreliosis in order to be counted and surveillance reports.

The most current report from the EU Commission regarding the LB incidence in Europe was published in 2008 for the years 1996 to 2005 by the Health and Consumers Directorate-General of Directorate C Public Health and Risk Assessment [51]. The report's surveillance data has two fundamental errors:

Under reporting: Many countries did not report data, reported intermittently or provided data that represented a small proportion of actual cases. For example, the data for Germany includes only two years (1998 and 1999) with near 1400 cases each year. In contrast, a study based on insurance claims gave an

© Copyright 2018. Global Network on Institutional Discrimination and
Ad Hoc Committee for Health Equity in ICD11 Borreliosis Codes. All Rights Reserved

estimate of 242 cases per 100,000 population for 2004 equivalent to an incidence of 214,000 cases for that year, suggesting the majority of diagnosed cases were not reported [52].

Calculation error: The total number of cases from some reporting European Union countries were applied to the total population of all 27 countries. *In contrast*, a calculation that uses the populations from countries that reported cases finds the LB incidence to be 19.7 cases per 100,000 for 2005 compared to the 4.1 cases per 100,000 published in the report. This makes for an almost five-fold under-reporting of cases [6].

Based on the US Centers for Disease Control and Prevention's (CDC) conservative estimate of annual LB infection in the USA, their 2017 article on persistent infection [53] and their 2006 study on the cost of Lyme borreliosis disease, the roughly 380,000 new LB infections each year cost the USA more than 4.09 billion dollars annually [54].

> In 2014, the NIH had a larger budget for headaches than for Lyme borreliosis, the fastest-growing infectious disease in America.

Since 2013, in the USA alone, there are an estimated 380,000 new annual Lyme borreliosis cases —more cases than breast cancer and more than six times the number of new HIV/AIDS cases.

Between 2013 and 2016, the CDC and National Institutes of Health (NIH) allocations for these illnesses ranged from approximately 20 million dollars a year for Lyme borreliosis, compared to over 650 million a year for breast cancer and nearly three billion dollars per year on HIV/AIDS.

II.4. Global Role of the Infectious Diseases Society of America (IDSA)

The IDSA's presents itself as a medical society. According to its website, the IDSA is also devoted to shaping policies and legislation globally regarding 'antimicrobial resistance, immunization, infection prevention and control, HIV/AIDS, tuberculosis, public health emergencies and other ID issues.' The IDSA has implemented an international strategy to maintain their views on Lyme borreliosis and assist their European colleagues in maintaining market dominance [55].

The following information provides details regarding the web of relationships and affiliations that set the European bias in favor of IDSA's opinions. According to European medical and scientific professionals, the IDSA favored the creation of a

---

[6] Faults in surveillance data and calculations provided by Michael Cook, engineer.

© Copyright 2018. Global Network on Institutional Discrimination and
Ad Hoc Committee for Health Equity in ICD11 Borreliosis Codes. All Rights Reserved

European Union Concerted Action on Lyme Borreliosis (EUCALB). Throughout Europe, including the Western, Eastern and Northern regions, EUCALB has maintained significant control or influence over the medical societies and the national reference centers for Lyme borreliosis.

EUCALB's views on LB have been widely promoted. This has led to the credibility and integrity of EUCALB's recommendations regarding LB to be widely questioned by medical and scientific professionals across Europe. For example, in a 2007 Elsevier publication of 'Medicine and Infectious Diseases' (Médecine et maladies infectieuses 2007) EUCALB recommended that European Union countries use a control group within a geographical area and limit their confirmations of LB infection to 'at most five percent' —*regardless of the actual numbers or percentage of LB infections* [56].

Recently, perhaps in response to a 2017 antitrust lawsuit filed against the IDSA, the website of EUCALB disappeared, however, the IDSA bias continues.

Currently, in most of Europe the LB public health messaging, treatment and research agenda is driven by the European Society of Clinical Microbiology and Infectious Diseases' (ESCMID) Study Group for Lyme Borreliosis (ESGBOR). ESGBOR has representation from every major university concerned with infectious diseases and many of these professors advise their governments on LB policy and practices. For example, as of 2017, the point person for ESGBOR is Ram Dessau of Slagelse, Denmark.

All three of the current ESGBOR Executive Committee —Chairperson Ram B. Dessau (Denmark) Secretary Tobias Rupprecht, (Germany) and Treasurer Gerold Stanek (Austria)— echo IDSA Lyme opinions and Stanek co-authored the 2006 IDSA Lyme Guidelines. The ESGBOR Executive Committee plays a role in screening of all new members and therefore can ensure the IDSA bias of the ESGBOR Study Group.

According to a 2010 presentation by Susan O'Connell, the former manager of the Lyme Disease Reference Laboratory at Southampton, there is overall agreement among guidelines promoted by certain medical societies in eleven European countries [57]. Under the Findings O'Connell states, "These recommendations, independently developed by a wide range of European experts in infectious diseases and other specialties, are similar to those of the IDSA."

In her acknowledgements O'Connell is "most grateful" to IDSA 2006 Lyme Guidelines' authors John Halperin, Gary

> During O'Connell's management of the Lyme Disease Reference Laboratory at Southampton UK, investigations uncovered multiple violations —the laboratory was closed in 2012.

21

© Copyright 2018. Global Network on Institutional Discrimination and
Ad Hoc Committee for Health Equity in ICD11 Borreliosis Codes. All Rights Reserved

Wormser, and Gerold Stanek and ESGBOR Executive Committee's Chairperson Ram Dessau.

For many years, Ram Dessau has been a key spokesperson defending the legitimacy and reliability of the Danish government's recommended serology tests for Lyme borreliosis. The recommended serology tests show 40 percent or less accuracy for females and more females than males are seronegative in these tests [58] [59]. Women who are seronegative for LB, even though they exhibit symptoms fully consistent with the disease, are often then denied treatment.

Dessau ignores the ECDC 2016 reports warning about the calibration of serologic tests and ignores the meta-analysis on Lyme serology published in 2016 by Cook and Puri [45].

A poignant example of the harm caused by this messaging by Dessau is Tabitha Nielsen, a desperately ill young Danish mother, who was denied LB treatment because her LB serology test was negative. She was subsequently diagnosed with LB clinically by a specialist, supported by the result of a different laboratory test, for which the test result provided laboratory evidence of infection with *Borrelia* and additional tick-borne infections.

Such tests are not included among those serological tests recommended by the IDSA and many State Actors, including the Danish, Dutch and US government, have all attacked such tests. Nevertheless, Tabitha's health improved significantly while under LB and co-infections treatment.

While Tabitha was under LB treatment, the Danish government's TV2 documentary 'Cheating or Borrelia' was aired in Denmark. Dessau was interviewed by TV2 the day following the release of the documentary in Denmark. He denounced the validity of tests not recommended by the Danish government or not provided by Danish laboratories —even though those laboratories and tests met all standards set by other member States of the European Union.

The Danish government's TV2 documentary and Dessau's opinion destroyed the funding support for Tabitha's LB treatment, making it impossible for her to afford ongoing treatment. This young mother is now in the process of dying from Lyme and co-infections.

The IDSA also uses a chat forum to send out news and alerts to all the members. At times this chat forum has been used to send out misinformation regarding 'incidents with Lyme patients' and LB protocols that have met internationally accepted standards and yet differ from the IDSA protocols.

© Copyright 2018. Global Network on Institutional Discrimination and
Ad Hoc Committee for Health Equity in ICD11 Borreliosis Codes. All Rights Reserved

On July 5, 2003, a 20-year-old woman in British Columbia, Canada died.

Within 48 hours and 3000 miles away, a patient in Nova Scotia, Canada, was told that 'fake Lyme diagnoses were killing people and that a girl in British Columbia has just died from the anaphylactic shock from unnecessary Lyme treatment' and that her doctor would not treat her Lyme infection.

In fact, she died from a nursing error and the inquiry confirmed this finding.

Nevertheless, the false story was perpetuated and even presented to the Canadian Parliament where it was publicly corrected by defenders of LB patients' human rights.

These misinforming alerts can result in immediate denial of treatment options for patients and wrongful defamation of practitioners who do not follow IDSA guidelines.

In Canada, the IDSA maintains their influence through private medical societies such as the Association of Medical Microbiology and Infectious Disease of Canada (AMMI) whose membership includes private medical professionals, and tax-payer salaried persons with positions of great influence in various levels of government. AMMI members are frequently called upon by insurers and government funded worker's compensation boards to review claims for coverage made by individuals for Lyme disease, both for disability coverage and drug coverage. These claims made by those individuals are then routinely denied.

A Freedom of Information request in Canada reveals the enmeshed relationship between the Canadian government and the IDSA.

Robbin Lindsay is a federal employee of the National Microbiology Laboratory under the Infectious Disease Prevention and Control Branch of the Public Health Agency of Canada. Todd Hatchette is the President of AMMI —the IDSA's sister organization in Canada— and Bill Bowie is the past president of AMMI. Most AMMI members are also IDSA members. Hatchett and Bowie are on provincial government dole for (at least) portions of their salaries.

On February 19, 2017, Lindsay, Hatchette and Bowie had email discussions regarding going to the CDC and Gary Wormser for clarification as to why the IDSA guidelines had been removed from the US federal National Guidelines Clearinghouse. They then discussed a competing medical society known as the International Lyme and Associated Diseases Society (ILADS). In this correspondence Lindsay states, "good grief, we are not following ILADS under any circumstances" and misrepresents both the ILADS process for guidelines development and composition of group that authored the ILADS Guidelines. Lindsay states, "no idea how the ILADS one [guidelines] would pass ... when they are based on input from three people."

© Copyright 2018. Global Network on Institutional Discrimination and
Ad Hoc Committee for Health Equity in ICD11 Borreliosis Codes. All Rights Reserved

In this case, one government staffer is deciding —*for all Canadians*— that the IOM approved ILADS clinical practice guidelines will never be seen by Canadian doctors or patients. ***This action by a State Actor obstructs both access to treatment options and informed consent.***

This 'coordination of message' from country to country among IDSA affiliates circumvents external oversight and governmental requirements for accountability and transparency in addition to promoting human rights violations.

II.4.1. IDSA Falsely Accuses Competitor of Making Death Threats

> "Their important work notwithstanding, defenders are
> increasingly subject to attacks by States and business-enterprises.
> Such attacks have taken place in all sectors and all regions."
> —Michel Forst, Special Rapporteur on the
> situation of human rights defenders.
> UN General Assembly in October 2017

On Wednesday, October 26, 2011, Professor Åse Bengaard Andersen, Chairman of the Danish Society for Infectious Medicine Location opened an international conference on the subject of further training for Danish doctors regarding Lyme Borreliosis [7]. German, Swedish, American (USA) and Danish professionals presented to the audience.

In the afternoon of October 26, Dr. Johan S. Bakken presented on 'Lyme Borreliosis: Scientific evidence and political consequences following the 2006 IDSA Guidelines.' Dr. Bakken is a consultant in infectious diseases at St. Luke's Hospital and a clinical associate professor at the University of Minnesota Medical School Duluth[8]. Dr. Bakken served as chair of the IDSA's State and Regional Societies Board and became the President of the IDSA in 2016.

Bakken has served on the IDSA Diagnostics Task Force, which examines the research, development, approval, manufacture, regulation and uptake of

---

[7] The 'Doctor Training on Borreliosis' conference was held in Auditorium 1 of Rigshospitalet in Copenhagen Denmark. The meeting was funded by the Organization of Medical Sciences companies and specialist companies in Clinical Microbiology, Infectious Medicine and Neurology (Mødet er finansieret af Organisationen af Lægevidenskabelige selskaber og specialeselskaberne i Klinisk Mikrobiologi, Infektionsmedicin og Neurologi).

[8] Dr. Johan Bakken graduated from the University of Washington (UW) School of Medicine in 1972. He completed an internship in internal medicine at the University of California Los Angeles and subsequent residencies in internal medicine at UW and the Lillehammer Regional Hospital in Norway. Dr. Bakken did his fellowship in ID at the University of Oslo, Norway, and completed a two-year postdoctoral fellowship in microbiology at Creighton University, Omaha, Nebraska in 1987.

24

© Copyright 2018. Global Network on Institutional Discrimination and
Ad Hoc Committee for Health Equity in ICD11 Borreliosis Codes. All Rights Reserved

This international conference had ten sessions.

Nine were devoted to medical and scientific presentations.

One session was devoted to defaming a medical society whose LB treatment guidelines meet the IOM's 2011 internationally accepted standards for clinical practice guidelines and evidence-based medicine.

infectious diseases diagnostics and was a contributor to the 2006 IDSA guidelines for Lyme borreliosis

His recent publications include the 2011 Antiscience and ethical concerns associated with advocacy of Lyme disease [60]. This article has received criticism from many countries and professionals in the field of medicine and science and has been the object of formal complaints to the US government [61].

As noted, the IDSA has a global strategy and network in place to collaborate on any number of infectious diseases and other concerns for ID specialists. Therefore, it is understandable the IDSA spends considerable resources to ensure up-to-date medical information is shared with their colleagues in other countries.

However, Bakken's presentation had little to do with the 'scientific evidence and political consequences following the 2006 IDSA Guidelines'. His presentation largely focused on discrediting a medical society known as International Lyme and Associated Diseases Society (ILADS). ILADS has clinical practice guidelines for Lyme borreliosis (LB) and other tick-borne diseases that differ from those of the IDSA.

The main differences are that ILADS recognizes that the standard two-tiered serology tests for LB are very unreliable [62] [45], LB infections can persist after a short course of antibiotics and ILADS will apply antimicrobial therapies based upon patient response. In addition, the ILADS guidelines conform to the IOM guidelines standards, but those of the IDSA, which are five years older, do not.

Bakken's PowerPoint presentation included many false, defamatory and libelous statements, including "ILADS members have resorted to harassment and death threats". Bakken cited the 2011 Antiscience and ethical concerns associated with advocacy of Lyme

A May 2017 PowerPoint presentation to a University of Toronto class reunion by Dr. Art Weinstein largely focused on LB patients, advocates and the doctors who treat persistent cases of LB.

He made derogatory and slanderous statements against these groups, in addition to the false statements in his presentation.

Weinstein is a US based rheumatologist with long ties to IDSA, including being a contributor to their Lyme Guidelines.

© Copyright 2018. Global Network on Institutional Discrimination and Ad Hoc Committee for Health Equity in ICD11 Borreliosis Codes. All Rights Reserved

disease article to support his statements [60]. However, these fabrications are not supported by the 2011 article he co-authored.

> "ILADS members have resorted to harassment and death threats"
> — PowerPoint Presentation Copenhagen

Why would Bakken, a man with decades invested in building his professional profile and credibility, resort to such self-incriminating and extreme behavior?

It is true there is a lack of consensus regarding the nature of these infections —Lyme borreliosis, Lyme-like borrelial infection as found in Australia and relapsing fever borreliosis— and how best to treat these patients.

However, attacks such as those documented in this Copenhagen conference used defamation, slander and libel rather than rely on scientific and medical arguments.

"It is not essential for a human rights defender to be correct in his or her arguments in order to be a genuine defender. The critical test is whether or not the person is defending a human right."
—OHCR

As previously noted, the fact remains that ILADS treatment guidelines meet internationally accepted standards. For this reason alone, **all LB patients, like any other patient group, should have their right to informed consent honored and, like any other patient group, should be able to choose among treatment options.**

II.4.2. IDSA Hinders Global Response to Lyme Borreliosis

The published viewpoint of the IDSA is that "Lyme is a mild illness, difficult to acquire, simple to diagnose and easy to treat".

They support diagnosis based upon a "two-tier" serologic testing scheme that has a published sensitivity of only 50 percent [62]. It is routine for manufacturers of these tests to include warnings that a negative test result does not mean the patient does not have Lyme. One meta-analysis publication showed the LB serology tests miss 500 times more cases compared to the two-stage HIV testing [45].

The IDSA gives no weight to clinical judgement in diagnosis nor have they accepted currently available, more accurate laboratory methods. Their treatment

26

© Copyright 2018. Global Network on Institutional Discrimination and
Ad Hoc Committee for Health Equity in ICD11 Borreliosis Codes. All Rights Reserved

recommendations are highly restrictive. For nearly all cases of infection, including patients who have been severely ill for many years, they advocate a "one size fits all" treatment strategy of low doses of oral antibiotics and restrict treatment duration to two to four weeks.

These restrictive views are not supported by peer reviewed published scientific literature. Many publications have documented the ability of *Borrelia* to alter their metabolism and morphology to evade host defenses and antibiotic therapy. Many more publications have conclusively documented the persistence of living *Borrelia* in previously treated animals and in previously treated humans.

In these cases of treatment failure, regimens were designed to mirror regimens advocated by the IDSA. These cases collectively document failure of the IDSA-recommended, simple, low dose and arbitrarily curtailed treatment regimens. In contrast, there is widespread experience by clinicians worldwide that a greatly improved rate of treatment success can be achieved if treatments are individualized to each patient's needs, and that includes repeated or more prolonged treatments with antibiotics if necessary.

In addition, the IDSA ignores that a Lyme patient can be co-infected with other tick-borne pathogens despite ample published evidence of the existence of co-infections in ticks, animals and humans. They do not address clinical presentation, diagnosis or treatment for these coinfected individuals.

II.5. IDSA in the USA

ID specialists have indispensable roles when it comes to national security threats from disease-causing microorganisms, whether natural or intentional in origin. These essential ID activities include the research and development of vaccines, drugs, therapies, and diagnostic tools for public health medical emergencies and acting as first responders to microbial threats.

The threat of epidemics from emerging infectious diseases such as Ebola and Zika and increasing bioterrorism threats have amplified recognition of the essential role ID specialists play in US and global health and welfare.

Since 1999, the IDSA has grown from 3,000 members to over 10,000 with international members throughout the world. IDSA members receive a significant portion of US government dollars for research regarding HIV, Hepatitis C, emerging microbial threats, bioterrorist threats of a microbial nature, the development of

© Copyright 2018. Global Network on Institutional Discrimination and
Ad Hoc Committee for Health Equity in ICD11 Borreliosis Codes. All Rights Reserved

vaccines, new antibiotics for drug resistant strains and diagnostic tools for public health emergencies.

IDSA members and their institutions often partner with the most powerful pharmaceutical companies in the world when undertaking these research and development (R&D) efforts. These pharmaceutical companies, known as Big Pharma, outspend all other special interest groups by hundreds of millions of dollars every year in their efforts to shape USA and international legislation and policy regarding healthcare.

Members of the IDSA hold key positions at medical journals, research institutions, and institutions of higher learning. Furthermore, the IDSA is deeply involved with numerous federal Health and Human Services (HHS) Agency programs, the umbrella organization for the CDC, the NIH and the Food and Drug Administration (FDA). IDSA members also submit patents in tandem with the NIH and CDC.

The IDSA has a significant advisory role for the Department of Defense (DOD) and routinely partners with the DOD on military and civilian health concerns. The IDSA is also represented in every major governmental and private sector decision-making entity related to infectious diseases, antibiotic stewardship, vaccines and so forth.

In the USA and many other countries, the IDSA has influenced how State Actors, medical societies and health systems respond to the Lyme and relapsing fever pandemic.

The CDC has ignored legislative language and directives to advance Lyme science, diagnostic and treatments detailed in the

---

Borrelia Grants to IDSA

In the US, between 2007-2016, approximately 950 government grants for 'Borrelia' were awarded. The authors of the 2006 IDSA Lyme Guideline's institutions received approximately two thirds more of these grants than other institutions.

On record with US Congressional offices are the 32 million dollars of NIH grants that have supported articles that attack those concerned and affected by complicated and persistent cases of Lyme disease. These articles:
- fail to meet their stated grant objectives
- show research misconduct, e.g. fabricate findings such as LB patients with persistent and complicated LB do not have infection or biological illness but suffer from psychiatric conditions — the psychiatric conditions have been repudiated by the American Psychiatric Association
- research methodology often fails basic quality standards, e.g. ignores substantial body of peer reviewed studies showing evidence of persistent LB infection
- defame and libel patients with complicated and persistent forms of LB and their human rights defenders

Their authors include authors of the 2006 IDSA Lyme Guidelines.

© Copyright 2018. Global Network on Institutional Discrimination and
Ad Hoc Committee for Health Equity in ICD11 Borreliosis Codes. All Rights Reserved

2002, 2010 and 2015 HHS Appropriations Bills to advance Lyme borreliosis science, diagnostic and treatments.

"In fiscal year 2000 the inventors of NIH intramural technologies received, as a group, 13.5 percent of total NIH royalty revenue, and 28 NIH inventors currently receive the maximum $150,000 annual royalty"

In accordance with the US Bayh-Dole Act, "the NIH distributes the royalty income in accordance with federal law and NIH policy. By law, federal inventors must receive the first $2,000 of income received by the agency and at least 15 percent thereafter, up to a maximum of $150,000 per year in royalties from all licensed technologies in which they are inventors...[63]

The IDSA also advocates to shape economic returns and financial opportunities for their membership, such as in their lobbying of legislation and policies. The topics covered for these financial opportunities include 'ID access and reimbursement, antimicrobial resistance, infection prevention and control, immunizations and vaccines, emerging infections and biothreats, research and infrastructure, global health, workforce and training, federal funding and diagnostics' [64].

The IDSA also implements strategies to ensure market dominance by discrediting their competitors. For example, bogus complaints filed by IDSA members against competing, non-IDSA physicians have precipitated disciplinary investigations by state health departments. In those cases involving LB, nearly all of the investigations were closed without action.

As a direct result of the capricious actions of the IDSA, non-IDSA health care providers and patients have sought assistance through legislative action to protect their rights. There are now more than 25 states to date that have passed or amended laws to ensure:

- LB patients have access to health care providers and treatment options that meet the 2011 IOM standards
- medical practitioners/human rights defenders can provide such care without harassment and penalty and loss of license
- patients are properly informed of the unreliability of the recommended serology tests as in 'a negative serology test does not mean you do not have Lyme borreliosis infection' [45]

Such laws provide limited protections, but alarmingly, nothing is being done by State Actors to curtail the unethical and anticompetitive practices of the IDSA.

© Copyright 2018. Global Network on Institutional Discrimination and
Ad Hoc Committee for Health Equity in ICD11 Borreliosis Codes. All Rights Reserved

In response to these legislative changes, the IDSA has been implementing an elaborate USA political strategy that ignores the science and medical knowledge regarding persistent and complicated LB, (see <u>Lyme Disease and State Policy</u>

<u>Primer for State Legislators-</u> Updated August 2016) and falsely claim that their competitors' practices are dangerous [64] [65].

Furthermore, the IDSA and their affiliates are implementing such tactics globally.

II.5.1. IDSA's Ethical and Legal Complications

In the case of Lyme borreliosis, there are IDSA members with a long-documented history of conflicts of interests (COI). These COIs appear to interfere with advances in diagnostic technologies and are implicated in the denial of insurance coverage for LB patients living with persistent and complicated cases.

The medical guidelines developed by a small subgroup of IDSA members explicitly rejects the use of direct detection diagnostic tests, such as polymerase chain reaction (PCR) for the diagnosis of Lyme disease. Such tests are a powerful means of diagnosis for various *Borrelia* species and other bacteria or parasites responsible for coinfections, particularly early in the infection when serological tests will be negative regardless of the infection status.

In 2011, the IOM formed a Committee on Standards for Developing Trustworthy Clinical Practice Guidelines (CPGs) and developed and published <u>Clinical Practice Guidelines We Can Trust</u> [66]. These 2011 IOM guidelines detailed the many reasons why CPGs need to be trustworthy and evidence-based [67].

In Chapter Three of the publication, the committee noted that many CPGs lack transparency regarding their development methodologies and that such methods varied significantly among the CPG developers, e.g. the roles of independent review and consensus were unclear and the links between CPGs and evidence was often inconsistent or lacking.

As case study to illustrate some of these shortcomings, the committee chose the 2006 IDSA Lyme Guidelines that is currently the 'template' for LB guidelines in many countries. The IDSA case study (found on page 56, BOX 3-1) details the lack of transparency regarding development methodologies and how the lack of recognition of and treatments for chronic LB prompted concern over the quality of evidence supporting the CPG development.

© Copyright 2018. Global Network on Institutional Discrimination and
Ad Hoc Committee for Health Equity in ICD11 Borreliosis Codes. All Rights Reserved

The case study notes COIs and the selection of guideline review committee members, e.g. some CPG authors were expert witnesses in legal proceedings related to LB or expert witness in LB malpractice cases initiated by health insurance companies against doctors who treat chronic LB and LB with coinfections. The lack of an independent review of the draft CPGs and lack of patient consultation was noted.

US Bayh-Dole Act

The federal laws for collaborating and benefiting from patents was radically transformed by the US Bayh-Dole Act. Findings from a 2012 report on the Bayh-Dole Act by the Congressional Research Service include [68]:

> "... collaboration may provide increased opportunities for conflicts of interest, redirection of research, less openness in sharing of scientific discovery, and a greater emphasis on applied rather than basic research"

Passed in 1980, the Act created a uniform patent policy among the many federal agencies to fund research with small businesses and non-profit organizations, including universities and to retain titles to inventions made under federally-funded research programs. Non-profits, including universities, and small businesses may elect to retain title to innovations developed under federally-funded research programs. Furthermore, anyone who is an inventor or assignee of a patent receives royalty payments from anyone licensed to utilize the technology patented. Other findings from the 2012 report state:

> "Additional concerns have been expressed, particularly in relation to the pharmaceutical and biotechnology industries, that the government and the public are not receiving benefits commensurate with the federal contribution to the initial research and development."
> The government plays a role in potentially "creating an unfair advantage for one company over another..."

> "The government receives a significant payback through taxes on profits"

> [paraphrased] '...under the Bayh-Dole Act, pharmaceuticals and biotechnology companies are receiving too many benefits at the expense of the public'

The issues identified in the 2012 report are readily found in the IDSA behaviors surrounding LB patents and clinical practice guidelines for LB. For example, the language for LB used by IDSA members and their affiliates in the hundreds of LB-

31

© Copyright 2018. Global Network on Institutional Discrimination and
Ad Hoc Committee for Health Equity in ICD11 Borreliosis Codes. All Rights Reserved

related patents listed on US and European patent sites stand in sharp contrast to the LB characterized in the 2006 IDSA Lyme guidelines.

IDSA and their associates acknowledge a complex LB illness in their patent applications, however, they openly deny or minimize this information in published materials and public opinions [69]. In fact, the language in many of these patents directly oppose the claims and opinions making up the 2006 guidelines [69].

Patents Do Not Lie

2007 Lyme Patent Language from IDSA Lyme Guideline co-author Raymond J. Dattwyler [et al] in filed patent No. 7605248 <u>Recombinant constructs of *Borrelia burgdorferi*</u> [70]

The language in this patent states:

"Currently, Lyme Disease is treated with a range of antibiotics, e.g., tetracyclines, penicillin and cephalosporins. However, such treatment is not always successful in clearing the infection.

Treatment is often delayed due to improper diagnosis with the deleterious effect that the infection proceeds to a chronic condition, where treatment with antibiotics is often not useful."

"One of the factors contributing to delayed treatment is the lack of effective diagnostic tools."

Versus

The 2006 IDSA Lyme Guidelines claim:

LB is 'easily treated, easily cured'

LB infection is easily cleared with antibiotics

Two-tier testing process should be utilized, and for those patients who test negative in the ELISA model, that "no further testing" is necessary.

© Copyright 2018. Global Network on Institutional Discrimination and
Ad Hoc Committee for Health Equity in ICD11 Borreliosis Codes. All Rights Reserved

Much that is known about LB has been carefully omitted from publications. Nevertheless, over decades patent language has consistently revealed scientific support for LB's complexity and persistence [69]

For example, a 1988 vaccine patent against LB (patent 4721617) [71] by Russell C. Johnson, PhD, now Professor Emeritus, Department of Microbiology and Immunology, of the University of Minnesota (assignees the Regents of the University of Minnesota) stated:

- "The etiological agent of this disease is the spirochete *Borrelia burgdorferi*, which is primarily transmitted by Ixodes ticks...Ixodes dammini is the major vector of Lyme disease in Minnesota, Wisconsin, the northeastern United States and adjacent Canada...I. pacificus is the primary vector of this disease in the western United States, and in Europe the major vector of Lyme borreliosis is I. ricinus. The spirochete has also been found in deerflies, horseflies and mosquitoes."
- "As many as two-thirds of the people that become infected by this spirochete are unaware of the tick bite because of the painless bite and the small size (several mm) of the nymphal stage."
- "The early phase of the illness often consists of the ECM, headache, fatigue, muscle and joint aches, stiff neck and chills and fever. This phase of the disease may be followed by neurologic, joint or cardiac abnormalities. The chronic forms of the disease such as arthritis (joint involvement), acrodermatitis chronica atrophicans (skin involvement), and Bannwart's syndrome (neurological involvement) may last for months to years and are associated with the persistence of the spirochete."
- "A case of maternal-fetal transmission of B. burgdorferi resulting in neonatal death has been reported."
- "For every symptomatic infection, there is at least one asymptomatic infection. Lyme disease is presently the most commonly reported tick-borne disease in the United States."
- "The infection may be treated at any time with antibiotics such as penicillin, erythromycin, tetracycline, and ceftriaxone."
- "Once infection has occurred, however, the drugs may not purge the host of the spirochete but may only act to control the chronic forms of the disease. Complications such as arthritis and fatigue may continue for several years after diagnosis and treatment."

The CDC and NIH both promote the 2006 IDSA Lyme guidelines. It is a violation of federal law for any US Agency to show preferential treatment for a private entity or 'give the appearance' of showing preferential treatment. This federal law was put in place to prevent government corruption and the appearance of corruption.

© Copyright 2018. Global Network on Institutional Discrimination and
Ad Hoc Committee for Health Equity in ICD11 Borreliosis Codes. All Rights Reserved

Antitrust Lawsuit Against the IDSA

On November 10, 2017, a group of LB patients filed a federal antitrust lawsuit in the U.S. District Court for the Eastern District of Texas, Texarkana Division - Case 5:17-cv-00190-RWS.

The patients allege that major health insurers are denying coverage for LB treatments based on factitious guidelines that were established by their paid IDSA consultants [72].

This preferential treatment by the CDC undermines free and fair market competition with non-IDSA private entities and smacks of corruption. Regardless, from 2006 until December 1, 2017, the CDC has actively promoted only the 2006 IDSA Lyme guidelines, even though there were other, more current guidelines that met the standards of the time.

Following an antitrust lawsuit filed against the IDSA in November 2017; the CDC website stopped their overt preferential promotion of the 2006 IDSA guidelines.

It should be noted that many CDC officials are members of the IDSA —including those responsible for LB and other TBDs.

However, the CDC website still describes the IDSA treatment regimen and directs the reader to an NIH website which then directs MedlinePlus Lyme Disease site (link is external); this direct is to the 2006 IDSA Lyme Guidelines [9].

Certain 2006 IDSA guideline authors have had special relationships with senior HHS officials responsible for LB policy and research grants. In March 2008, in violation of federal law [73], two government officials colluded with the authors to undermine the passing of the Maryland Lyme Disease Public Awareness Bill HB 838 [74].

There have been numerous formal complaints made by individuals and advocacy groups to the HHS Office of the General Counsel and the Ethics Division, the Office of the Inspector General and the CDC regarding this preferential treatment and collusion. It does not appear that any of the government officials responsible for these actions suffered any consequences.

From the 1990s thru 2007, 202 patents on Lyme borrelioses were accumulated by those IDSA member associated with the IDSA Lyme clinical practice guidelines development and their affiliates in government and other private entities [69].

---

[9] CDC website (www.cdc.gov/lyme/treatment/index.html) to NIH link (www.niaid.nih.gov/diseases-conditions/lyme-disease) where states: "To learn about risk factors for Lyme Disease and current prevention and treatment strategies visit the MedlinePlus Lyme Disease site (link is external)." Viewed February 8, 2018

34

© Copyright 2018. Global Network on Institutional Discrimination and
Ad Hoc Committee for Health Equity in ICD11 Borreliosis Codes. All Rights Reserved

IDSA Members and Organizations Associated with IDSA Holding LB-Related Patents in 2007 [69]	
1. *Raymond J. Dattwyler [US & foreign patents] 2. *Stephen Dumler [US Patents] 3. Alan Barbour [US & foreign patents] 4. Stanley Stein and Hoffman-Laroche 5. Ira Schwartz & New York Medical College (NYMC) 6. Avant Immunotherapeutics 7. Aventis Pasteur 8. Baxter → *Susan O'Connell, IDSA promoter worked for Baxter* 9. Becton-Dickinson 10. Boston Medical Center Corp. 11. Biomerieux 12. Cambridge Biotech 13. CDC 14. Columbia University 15. Immunetics 16. Johns Hopkins University 17. Mayo Clinic 18. Medimmune and Aventis, Medimmune 20. University of Minnesota *co-authors undisclosed COIs during the 2006 IDSA Lyme Guidelines development*	21. NIH/National Institute of Allergies and Infectious Diseases (NIAID) 22. NYMC 23. Pasteur Merieux/Connaught 24. Rx Technologies 25. SmithKline Beecham (under GlaxoSmith Kline) → *Danish Dr. Court Pedersen advises the Danish government and medical practitioners on LB and is supported by GlaxoSmithKline* 26. State of Rhode Island 27. Stony Brook University (SUNY) 28. Texas A&M University 29. Tufts New England Medical Center 30. Tufts US patents with Paratech and GlaxoSmithKline 31. Tulane University 32. University of California 33. University of Connecticut 34. US Army/US DHHS 35. Vical Inc. 36. Viro Dynamics 37. Yale University & Yale's Office of Cooperative Research Patents

III.   The Defenders of Lyme and Relapsing Fever Borreliosis Patients

"What is most important in characterizing a person as a human rights defender is not the person's title or the name of the organization he or she works for, but rather the human rights character of the work undertaken [11]."
—UN Office of the High Commissioner for Human Rights (OHCR)

35

© Copyright 2018. Global Network on Institutional Discrimination and
Ad Hoc Committee for Health Equity in ICD11 Borreliosis Codes. All Rights Reserved

There are many categories of Human Rights Defenders for patients with Lyme or relapsing fever borreliosis. As noted, they include members of nongovernmental organizations, patient groups, government officials, elected officials, scientists, medical professionals, researchers and laboratory and clinic owners.

The very existence of this large and diverse group of interested and affected parties and the many hundreds of support groups that have appeared underscore not only the seriousness of this pandemic but also the outdated, incorrect and corrupted official stance on borrelioses in general and the harm inflicted on professionals and patients alike.

> The Special Rapporteur for the situation of defenders "has expressed concern for the situation of human rights defenders in all countries, including both emerging democracies and countries with long-established democratic institutions, practices and traditions [75]."

All of these types of defenders provide critical support to this patient community. There are nonprofit organizations such as the Canadian Lyme Disease Foundation (CanLyme) that 'is dedicated to raising awareness and promoting Lyme Disease research, education and treatment' and provides grants to medical/science research students and investigators. CanLyme also provides a literal lifeline to LB patients who have been rejected from healthcare systems across the globe. Anyone, anywhere in the world, can call the CanLyme phone number and receive answers directly from an informed advocate.

Generally speaking, few of the defenders from non-science and nonmedical nonprofits have come under attack by State actors. There are other kinds of defenders that do not appear to be under direct attack, such as lawyers who facilitate disability benefits for this patient group.

This report focuses on the defenders who routinely experience documented human rights violations as a result of 'acting in support of victims of human rights violations'. Those human rights defenders who routinely experience these violations are:

- Medical practitioners and owners of clinics who practice informed consent and provide treatment options, including those that meet the 2011 internationally accepted standards set by the Institute of Medicine.
- Medical practitioners who have each successfully treated hundreds to over ten thousand patients with persistent and complicated cases.
- Scientists and researchers demonstrating treatment failure from short-term antibiotic therapies as advocated by the IDSA and evidence of persistent infection following such therapies.

36

© Copyright 2018. Global Network on Institutional Discrimination and
Ad Hoc Committee for Health Equity in ICD11 Borreliosis Codes. All Rights Reserved

- Owners and professionals of laboratories that provide more accurate diagnostic tests than those that are recommended by the IDSA and its supporters —tests that can capture 'seronegative' antibody infections. These newer and more sensitive diagnostic assays include direct detection methods and serologic diagnostic tests that utilize a wider range of borreliosis strains than the IDSA-recommended serology tests. Such tests provide earlier and greater opportunity for this patient group to be correctly diagnosed and treated.
- Medical practitioners who have made clinical diagnosis of Lyme and/or relapsing fever borreliosis infections, then went on to treat with antimicrobial therapies that successfully minimized symptoms or halted the progression of 'incurable diseases' (previously misdiagnosed).
- Medical practitioners, scientists, researchers and laboratory owners who criticize government policies that ignore and obstruct access to treatment options that have met international standards for clinical practice guidelines.
- Medical practitioners, scientists, researchers and laboratory owners who testify in defense of others who support informed consent and access to treatment options.
- Medical practitioners, scientists, researchers and laboratory owners who are competing with patents and professionals who are benefiting from the mischaracterization that these infections are 'hard to catch, easy to diagnose and easy to cure'.
- Parents defending their rights to: prohibit the administration of medicine to a child against parents' wishes, to freedom from torture and cruel, inhuman and degrading treatment, freedom of association, participation in public policy, due process and remedy; and
  - ➢ their sick children's rights to: liberty and security of person, privacy and confidentiality, bodily integrity, the highest attainable standard of health, freedom from torture and cruel, inhuman and degrading treatment, nondiscrimination and equality and remedy.

The human rights defenders of Lyme and relapsing fever borreliosis patients highlighted in this report:

- have been consistently threatened with the loss of their professional licenses and livelihoods
- have had their livelihoods destroyed and licenses removed
- are routinely targeted for harassment, defamation, slander and libel
- are burdened with probationary measures that curtail their freedom of movement and assembly and their right to free speech and associational life
- experience false accusations, undue process and conviction

These violations have often targeted the human rights defenders themselves, as well as the organizations and mechanisms through which they work.

© Copyright 2018. Global Network on Institutional Discrimination and
Ad Hoc Committee for Health Equity in ICD11 Borreliosis Codes. All Rights Reserved

IV. The Nature of the Human Rights Violations Against the Defenders of Lyme and Relapsing Fever Borreliosis Patients

"Defenders are active in support of human rights [such as] the highest attainable standard of health [and] to non-discrimination. They sometimes address the rights of categories of persons [11]."

—OHCR

Lyme and relapsing fever borreliosis patients and their human rights defenders are treated by healthcare systems and State Actors in ways that contrast sharply with most patient groups suffering from complicated systemic infections and those who support their access to diagnosis and care.

These contrasts are confounding, disturbing and illuminating. In many countries, these discriminatory practices are linked to conflicts of interest and indicate corruption.

In most of these cases, State Actors (government) such as State health authorities, and State-appointed bodies such as Medical Boards, are the perpetrators of these violations.

Medical Boards are organizations run by medical doctors to oversee the functioning of their colleagues. Those medical board members who aggressively attack the defenders of LB patients have IDSA affiliations and/or are members of the IDSA.

> SR Michel Forst "is deeply concerned that these defenders are suffering attacks by business actors overpowering and silencing them, which exerts a chilling effect on their work. This worrying trend is compounded by a lack of State action in response to such attacks."
>
> —October 2017
> to UN General Assembly

The nature of the charges by the State Actors and State appointed bodies often do not specify LB diagnosis and treatment as the cause for harassment, spurious accusations, unfair trials and convictions. The sham charges against these human rights defenders typically fall into a few categories; examples follow in sections IV.1. – IV.4.

IV.1. Category One: 'Inadequate Record-Keeping'

Those practitioners known to provide care for persistent and complicated LB cases are often accused of 'inadequate' record-keeping and/or 'poor' communications. This allegation then allows actions by Medical Boards —wherein any infraction, no matter how minor and even if no patients were harmed, allows sanctions to be

© Copyright 2018. Global Network on Institutional Discrimination and
Ad Hoc Committee for Health Equity in ICD11 Borreliosis Codes. All Rights Reserved

imposed. These sanctions can include fines, monitoring paid for by the practitioner and onerous reporting, monitoring and probationary sentences.

The burdens of these probationary measures curtail the defenders' freedom of movement. For example, they may not be able to attend any number of scientific or medical conferences outside of the immediate area of their practice, state, province or country. In addition, they must seek legal counsel for the defense of their medical license, which causes significant financial burden.

Furthermore, such a charge may allow the Medical Boards and State medical authorities full access to confidential patient files. Here, the practitioner is not allowed to inform his patients that their medical records are under review. Alarmingly, this a violation of the patient's confidentiality in that their records must be released even if the patient objects.

In some cases, these 'inadequate record-keeping charges' are used as an intimidation tactic, to make the practitioner reluctant to continue to treat affected patients or to submit to pressure and reclassify the medical illness to a psychosomatic one. For example, a patient with cardiac complications from Lyme borreliosis may suddenly find their cardiac specialist becomes more concerned with making sure they take drugs for psychosomatic illness rather than be treated for biological cardiac problems. Instead of focusing on appropriate patient care, the investigation changed to emphasize record keeping.

IV.2. Category Two: 'Unnecessary Treatment'

Another common charge against defender practitioners is that their patients 'do not have tick-borne diseases' or 'do not have biological illness but instead suffer from psychosomatic illness' and thus any biological treatment is deemed 'not medically necessary'.

As noted in most governmental LB policies:
(1) Lyme borreliosis is a clinical diagnosis; and
(2) the recommended serology tests can be helpful in validating the clinical diagnosis, but they are not intended to overturn the clinical diagnosis.

Nevertheless, practitioners who appropriately diagnose and treat based upon clinical grounds are charged with violations if the patient does not have a positive serology test.

39

© Copyright 2018. Global Network on Institutional Discrimination and
Ad Hoc Committee for Health Equity in ICD11 Borreliosis Codes. All Rights Reserved

Furthermore, most State and State-appointed entities use for diagnosis the narrow case definition that was designed for LB surveillance and not for clinical diagnosis.

Surveillance case definitions are intentionally restrictive— for surveillance one wants strictly defined and confirmed cases and it is widely accepted that this will miss many cases. On the other hand, clinical case definitions recognize the severely limited accuracy of serologic blood tests and emphasize history and clinical presentation, among other factors, and put less weight on unreliable tests.

In fact, in the USA, the CDC website clearly states the LB case definition is to be used for surveillance and *not* for diagnosis. Yet despite this and the many hundreds of peer-reviewed publications that support clinical diagnoses, these State entities proceed with charges against those that do not use the surveillance definition for diagnosis.

Treatment of disseminated Lyme borreliosis is often difficult, as there are no tests or markers that can conclusively define the optimal duration and endpoint of treatment. Therapeutic decisions must be made on an ongoing and individualized basis because of the unique way each patient responds. Experienced clinicians recognize this and tailor treatment accordingly.

In contrast, State Actors and their agents adhere to the outdated and restrictive IDSA "one size fits all" treatment scheme. This entails treating all cases similarly and it includes an arbitrary cutoff of treatment after three to four weeks.

This practice results in up to half of all patients remaining symptomatic after this brief regimen and many scientific studies have shown that these

---

Overt Gender-based Discrimination Sponsored by State Actors

Multiple medical studies have shown the strong clinical bias to label women's health status, versus that of men, as being psychosomatic rather than biological in nature.

As noted, the recommended serology tests show 40 percent or less accuracy for females and more females than males show seronegative [46] [58].

Government-sponsored entities and articles have added to the LB gender bias by falsely portraying women suffering from persistent and complicated LB cases as 'having attention seeking behaviors', psychosomatic illness, lacking the judgment or strength of character to make informed medical choices on their own behalf and on behalf of their children, lacking capacity to manage stress, discomfort and everyday life [76] [77].

This creates dynamics wherein seronegative women are likely to be diagnosed as psychosomatic and not provided **needed medical care**.

© Copyright 2018. Global Network on Institutional Discrimination and
Ad Hoc Committee for Health Equity in ICD11 Borreliosis Codes. All Rights Reserved

infections can persist due to this inadequate treatment regimen. In such cases, their ongoing illness reflects treatment failure.

However, IDSA claims, without supporting evidence, that these patients are cured of the infection and any remaining symptoms remain are due to a 'post Lyme syndrome' —a condition that has never been demonstrated to exist. In contrast, in cancer care, if a tumor remains after a round of chemotherapy, the patient is not said to have 'post cancer syndrome' —the patient is retreated with a more prolonged or aggressive regimen.

Unfortunately, if a practitioner extends treatment for on-going LB symptoms, the practitioner may be accused of "overtreatment" even if the treatment was beneficial to the patient and may also face retaliation if they testify on behalf of patients' coverage for treatments. This retaliation may come from authorities related to child protection should they testify on behalf of ill children.

To note, many patients are coinfected with more than one tick-borne pathogen and antibiotic combinations are usually required to target the different infections. However, because the IDSA guidelines do not address coinfections, antibiotic combinations are not recommended by them. Treatment of coinfections is one more way that the practitioner can be charged. Usually these complaints against practitioners are made by health insurance companies that do not want to pay for more medications, or by competing doctors who follow the IDSA guidelines.

These sham charges ignore the accepted fact that LB is a clinical diagnosis and the many peer-reviewed publications that support this. These factitious charges also ignore the tens of thousands of documented clinical cases and the hundreds of cases cited in the peer reviewed literature that clearly document persistent infection, treatment failure, need for addressing coinfections and benefit of additional treatment beyond what the IDSA recommends.

IV.3. Category Three: Hypocrisy Regarding Antibiotic Use

Hypocrisy underscores the criticism against the defenders' antibiotic stewardship and their use of intravenous antimicrobial therapies.

Peripherally Inserted Central Catheter (PICC) lines and other intravenous (IV) technologies are routinely used in home infusions, hospital settings and private clinics to deliver antimicrobial therapies for many intractable or persistent infections. Occasionally these IV catheters become infected. The informed consent

© Copyright 2018. Global Network on Institutional Discrimination and
Ad Hoc Committee for Health Equity in ICD11 Borreliosis Codes. All Rights Reserved

of patients is a routine part of the process for proceeding with these interventions.

In the USA, the IDSA has lobbied to have open-ended home infusions therapies, including IV antimicrobials, for any number of infections to be covered by Medicare, Medicaid and insurance companies [78]. These therapies are indeed covered by many insurance companies.

The occasional infections arising from these IV therapies rarely result in investigations or punishments for the involved medical professionals [79] [80].

This is in part due to the fact such infections are considered a known and acceptable risk. "Venous access is one of the most basic yet critical components of patient care both in hospital and in ambulatory patient settings. Safe and reliable venous access is an important issue in daily practice..." [81] [79]

In contrast, the US, Canadian and Scandinavian medical practitioners who provide clinic and home-based IV therapies for their LB patients are routinely investigated and penalized. These investigations occur even without incidents of complications from the IV therapies.

Such investigations are often initiated by insurance companies to contain costs, or by doctors who follow the IDSA guidelines, and involve State Actors and State-appointed Actors, such as Medical Boards or 'Child Protection Services'.

© Copyright 2018. Global Network on Institutional Discrimination and
Ad Hoc Committee for Health Equity in ICD11 Borreliosis Codes. All Rights Reserved

IV.4. Superbugs and Antibiotic Stewardship

The IDSA has falsely indicated that LB patients are prone to developing 'superbugs' when given prolonged antibiotic therapy. Superbugs are bacteria that have developed resistance to antibiotics.

There is no scientific or medical basis for these statements as LB patients demonstrate no enhanced capacity or tendency over any other patient group for developing superbugs.

In addition, antibiotic stewardship practices for human use and animal use vary from country to country. In the USA, antibiotic stewardship practices are shaped very much by lobbying rather than scientific and medical consensus.

For example, antibiotic use in animal farming varies widely and its practices do not necessarily conform to 'stewardship practices' to conserve for human use.

> State policies supporting IDSA Lyme opinions are costly to patients and result in many turning to crowd funding to pay for treatment options that met international standards.
>
> In 2017 —numbers from the top five crowd funding sites (GoFundMe, Kickstarter, etc.) — commonly added up to approximately one million posts requesting funds for LB treatment and related travel.

In the US, roughly 75 percent of all antibiotics used are fed to farm animals [82]. The US Food and Drug Administration's (FDA) data shows that in 2015, 74 percent of antibiotics for farm animals was administered in their feed and 21 percent via the drinking water. Altogether, an estimated 95 percent of farm antibiotics are being used for mass medication. In 2011, total antibiotic use in human medicine was 3,290 tonnes of active ingredient, making the medically important antibiotics in food animals in the US approximately three times higher than human use [10].

The EU unit measure used for the size of livestock populations is the "Population Correction Unit" (PCU). Levels of antibiotic use vary significantly by farm animal species making it difficult to estimate the antibiotic use and adherence to stewardship practices. For example, pigs, poultry and veal calves tend to be intensively farmed and when they are intensively farmed they have very high antibiotic use whereas pasture-raised sheep and cattle tend to have much lower antibiotic use. However, there is no available published data on the PCU of livestock species.

---

[10] "These data do not include the further 5,785 tonnes of non-medically important antimicrobials (including 4,741 tonnes of the ionophore antibiotics) which are used in US farm animals." Farm antibiotic use in the United States August 2017. Alliance to Save our Antibiotics

© Copyright 2018. Global Network on Institutional Discrimination and
Ad Hoc Committee for Health Equity in ICD11 Borreliosis Codes. All Rights Reserved

V. How Violations Against Human Rights Defenders Harm Lyme and Relapsing Fever Borreliosis Patients

As noted, State health authorities and State-appointed bodies have actively restricted these defenders' right to speak and educate freely on the nature of Lyme and relapsing fever borreliosis. They have restricted the defenders' capacity to provide care to Lyme and relapsing fever borreliosis patients who seek their assistance. State actors and appointed bodies have prohibited these defenders from their full participation and representation in any number of associations and assemblies.

The nature and scale of reprisals committed against those who defend and provide access to diagnosis and treatment options for Lyme and relapsing fever borreliosis patients is well-documented in many countries including Canada, France, Belgium, Australia, the USA and Scandinavian countries. Regardless of these attacks, the actions taken by these human rights defenders are peaceful.

In these cases, State and State-appointed Actors manipulate legislation and authority —that theoretically conforms to international human rights law and medical ethics— with the result of obstructing:

- patient access to diagnosis provided by laboratories that meet the required local or national standards
- access to treatment options that meet internationally accepted standards
- access to educators (who are also defenders) with up-to-date medical and scientific knowledge regarding Lyme and relapsing fever borreliosis

Furthermore, in many cases these human rights defenders are the providers of clinical diagnosis and therapies that meet international standards.

In this way, the nature and scale of these reprisals against the human rights defenders is compounded into human rights violations against the patient groups. Human rights violations against the patient groups are recognized as humiliating, degrading, severe, life-threatening, and at times fatal.

Furthermore, such practices against the human rights defenders interfere with the Right to Health [83]; this is a fundamental right enshrined within the international human rights framework and consistent with the imperative of Availability, Accessibility, Acceptability, Quality (AAAQ) of care [84].

In effect, attacks on these human rights defenders obstruct access to diagnosis and care for hundreds of thousands across the globe. For example, medical

44

© Copyright 2018. Global Network on Institutional Discrimination and
Ad Hoc Committee for Health Equity in ICD11 Borreliosis Codes. All Rights Reserved

practitioners who have provided therapies for persistent and complicated cases of LB for more than one decade often have treated thousands of such patients. Therefore, every time an attack succeeds in removing one such medical practitioner, many thousands of patients may lose access to care.

The human rights violations against these defenders result in additional obstruction to patient diagnosis and care. Without treatment options, patients may consequently become debilitated, disabled, lose quality-of-life and productive capacity, experience bankruptcy, the destruction of their social support and family, have unnecessary pain and suffering and early death.

Prohibition of Internet Use

The internet is an invaluable tool for accessing information —including scientific and medical information.

In the UK, general practitioners may reject patients, including those with Lyme and other tickborne diseases, who admit to accessing medical information from the Internet.

VI.   Examples of the Situation of the Defenders

Section VI provides more characterizations and insight regarding their situation from the human rights defenders. Section VI also provides additional comparisons as to how these defenders are treated versus their peers who are not involved with persistent and complicated Lyme and relapsing fever borreliosis.[11]

VI.1. Comparisons of Penalties

There are striking differences between how State Actors interact with medical practitioners who limit their treatment according to the IDSA guidelines and those practitioners who recognize and treat persistent and complicated cases of LB and co-infections according to patient response. This pattern of distinctive discrimination extends to laboratory scientists.

VI.1.1. Canada

In Canada's most heavily populated province, Ontario, there are over 40,000 physicians. *Fewer than one percent* are ever investigated for alleged improper practice. However, of the physicians who became known to diagnose and treat LB based upon the clinical indications, they are approaching 100 percent who have been investigated and penalized.

---

[11] Some of the content of Section VI is drawn from interviews and therefore reflect a more conversational style.

© Copyright 2018. Global Network on Institutional Discrimination and
Ad Hoc Committee for Health Equity in ICD11 Borreliosis Codes. All Rights Reserved

For example, a very highly qualified specialist in Internal Medicine, Infectious Disease, and Medical Microbiology diagnosed and treated a patient for Lyme disease had a complaint registered against him, not from his patient, but from a neurologist who referred the patient to another Infectious Disease doctor [85].

According to the legal proceedings, as a result of his treatments, the specialist "began to wean the patient off the narcotics and psycho-affective drugs with which his symptoms were being treated because he felt that those medications were potentially harmful to the patient. The doctor reported that the patient's condition improved overall by more than 60 percent and that he was no longer bed-ridden."

Upon appeal... "The Board further found that the Committee reached an unreasonable decision to caution the Applicant [the Internal Medicine specialist] for failing to document the rationale and for not following the recommended guidelines for treatment of Lyme disease.

The Applicant's consultation letter to the patient's family physician, dated December 10, 2010, contained a detailed explanation of the treatment recommended."

The Internal Medicine specialist was right, he did not have to follow the Canada-wide imposed IDSA guidelines. Furthermore, he had explained his rationale for not using those guidelines to the family physician.

> In Canada alone, a petition launched in February 2017 in response to the release of the Canadian Federal Framework on Lyme Disease is currently at over 53,000 signatures.
>
> A nonprofit called LymeHope collected 2,700 personal letters from Canadians coast to coast documenting the immense harm and suffering from an over reliance on faulty testing, routine denial of access to testing, missed diagnosis and prohibition of treatment beyond an arbitrary two or three weeks.
>
> CanLyme collected many hundreds of similar video testimonials for the Canadian parliament.
>
> Similar exhaustive documentation is on record with State Actors in the US, UK, Australia and many European nations.

VI.1.2. Oregon, USA

Prior to becoming the Director of the Southern Oregon Community Care Organization (CCOs), Dr. James F. Calvert's license was under 'stipulated order'. While under stipulated order, a patient died under Calvert's care and his death resulted in another order [86]. While under this probation, Calvert was removed of liability. The Oregon Medical Board (OMB) then fully reinstated Calvert's medical license before he had begun the required remediation program put forth by the OMB.

© Copyright 2018. Global Network on Institutional Discrimination and
Ad Hoc Committee for Health Equity in ICD11 Borreliosis Codes. All Rights Reserved

This reinstatement came after the OMB documented Calvert's poor medical practices including his overuse and inappropriate use of opiates and other drugs within his patient population and misdiagnosis of multiple patients with rheumatological diseases.

For example, Calvert continued to treat his patient for lupus despite negative test results for lupus and despite the opinion by a Rheumatologist the patient did not have lupus. The treatment included opiates, marijuana, steroids and methotrexate and the patient almost died. Following his reinstatement, Calvert then became an employee of Oregon Health Authority as the Director of the Southern Oregon CCO. CCOs implement the Oregon Health Plan for low-income patients. Calvert continues to act as an expert witness for OMB on medical specialties for which he is untrained.

As CCO Director, Calvert has oversight on who gets treated by whom, and where. In this role, Calvert has been instrumental in obstructing access to medical care for patients suffering from LB and other tickborne diseases (TBDs). For example, a child from a low-income family had a history of tick bites, a positive serology test for LB and symptoms of Lyme arthritis, life threatening cardiac complications, and neurological complications that included severe systemic pain and excessive blinking. When the parents continued to question the Director regarding the lack of medical care for their child's Lyme infection, Calvert had the child reviewed by a neurologist who stated the lab testing was a possible false-positive as there was a lack of endemic *Borrelia* in the state. This statement ignores the tick collection exercises that have proven Lyme is present in Oregon and in the child's home region.

Follows IDSA 2006 Guidelines		Follows Treatment Guidelines that Meet the 2011 IOM Standards
In Oregon, a Dr. Calvert was put on probation for patient "death by negligence". While under probation, this doctor was allowed: • to treat patients • to hold an influential advisory role for the Oregon Department of health • testify against those doctors that treat patients with persistent and complicated LB and coinfections.	**versus**	In contrast to Calvert who is on probation for patient death by negligence, another Oregon doctor —known for treating complicated LB cases— was put on probation for 'poor record keeping' and has more restrictions than Dr. Calvert. These restrictions include: • no longer allowed to treat Lyme patients • no advising or testifying to the State government or legislators about Lyme borreliosis

© Copyright 2018. Global Network on Institutional Discrimination and
Ad Hoc Committee for Health Equity in ICD11 Borreliosis Codes. All Rights Reserved

Map of the distribution of the principal vectors of *B. burgdorferi* ss. in the United States 1907 through 1996 [87]

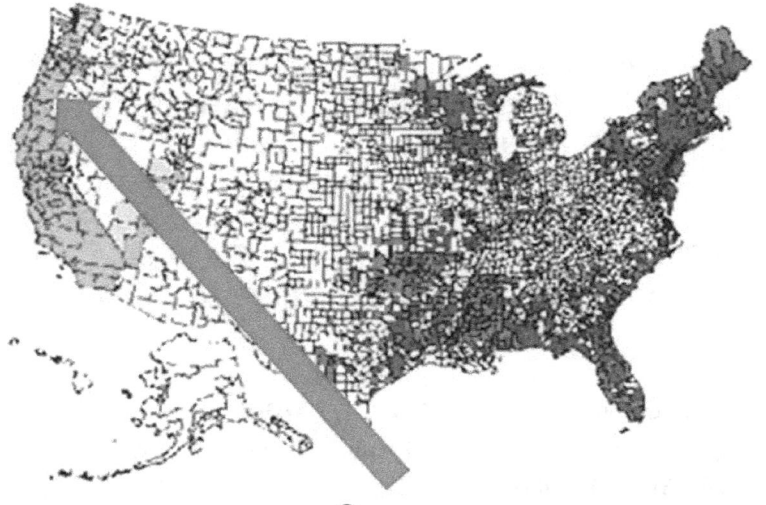

By-county distribution of the Lyme disease vectors Ixodes scapularis and Ixodes pacificus.

Red: established Ixodes scapularis
Blue: reported Ixodes scapularis
Green: established Ixodes pacificus
Yellow: reported Ixodes pacificus

Oregon

The Oregon Lyme Disease Network (OLDN), a local non-profit, provided both financial and letter writing support for the child's much needed medical care. Disabilities from Lyme disease and co-infections prevented the child from attending school for two years. OLDN wrote letters, attended Individualized Education Program (IEP) meetings and successfully advocated for home tutoring support.

VI.1.3. In Europe: Laboratories that Test for Lyme

Persecution and unfair treatment of clinicians have taken place in the UK. The governing body for doctors is the General Medical Council (GMC). The GMC considers complaints against doctors and can remove their license to practice. Complaints were lodged with the GMC against a number of doctors who treated Lyme disease. These were not from patients but from the manager of the Lyme Disease Reference Laboratory at Southampton, who has reported an interest in civil and criminal cases [88]. The manager of the Laboratory was Susan O'Connell, A member of the Ad Hoc International Lyme Group that included the authors of the 2006 IDSA Lyme Guidelines [89]. O'Connell's basic complaints were that 'the treated patients had received negative test results from her laboratory and so did not have Lyme disease'.

48

© Copyright 2018. Global Network on Institutional Discrimination and
Ad Hoc Committee for Health Equity in ICD11 Borreliosis Codes. All Rights Reserved

During O'Connell's management of the Lyme Disease Reference Laboratory, an audit of the quality management systems was triggered by patients tested at the laboratory [12]. In parallel, a second patient-led investigation identified many violations of test method procedures and these were confirmed during the UK Parliamentary and Health Services Ombudsman complaint process.

The audit and investigations led to the discovery of multiple issues and the laboratory was closed. O'Connell's laboratory was found to have falsely claimed an International Organization for Standardization (ISO) accreditation. An investigation by the UK Parliamentary and Health Services Ombudsman found many violations including:

- used a test certified only for use with blood serum for testing cerebrospinal fluid (CSF)
- modified the incubation time of the LB Western Blot test kit without validating for sensitivity and gave incorrect interpretation of Western Blot test results
- used a test kit specific for *Borrelia burgdorferi* B31 strain in Europe where other species are far more prevalent without validating the performance sensitivity
- failure to notify clinicians that the test was used off-label
- failure to follow the test kit manufacturer's instructions, e.g. calibration sheets were destroyed, and visual judgement used
- the laboratory recording system was so poor it resulted in misinterpretation by the Public Health England (PHE) and erroneous results submitted to patients during the complaint process

Promotes IDSA		Competes with IDSA
The UK laboratory was closed in 2012. O'Connell was 'retired' with a £40,000 bonus (55,523.60 US dollars). She then went to work for Baxter on the Lyme vaccine. Some 2006 IDSA Lyme Guideline authors were in business with Baxter.	**versus**	Viviane Schaller, a French biologist from Strasbourg, ran a lab that performed more sensitive Western Blot tests than the standard diagnostics. Schaller was condemned with a suspended prison sentence, more than 200,000 € (244,964 US dollars) in penalties and her lab was closed. A cassation appeal is now under examination.

---

[12] Information regarding the management issues of the Lyme Disease Reference Laboratory at Southampton provided by Michael Cook.

© Copyright 2018. Global Network on Institutional Discrimination and
Ad Hoc Committee for Health Equity in ICD11 Borreliosis Codes. All Rights Reserved

VI.1.4. Australia

To date no *B.burgdorferi sensu stricto* has been found in Australian ticks. However, Australians do travel to countries where LB is present and in Australia there are recognized borrelial infections and relapsing fever borreliosis that demonstrate 'Lyme-like' illness and symptoms.

These *Borrelia* species are not identical to *Borrelia* species that cause Lyme borreliosis, but it is widely known that other *Borrelia* cause human disease. Significantly, these "Lyme-like *Borrelia*" are different enough that they will not be detected by government-sanctioned LB serology tests.

SR Michel Forst, "Many testimonies unveiled the complicity of States, which tended to pursue cases brought by businesses against human rights defenders while ignoring cases reported by defenders against businesses"
—October 2017 to UN General Assembly

In the last six years, all Australian doctors known to treat LB and Lyme-like illness have been investigated. Compared to doctors not known for treating Lyme, these doctors are picked on for minor or imaginary breaches of medical conduct and the significance these breaches have been amplified to give larger punishments.

Not Known for Treating Lyme

- In 2005, Dr. Jayant of Patel Bundaberg Hospital was reprimanded and deregistered for 86 avoidable patient deaths. He had a minimal prison sentence and minor financial penalty.

- A Camberra-based orthopedic surgeon harmed 400 patients. After 12 years of patient complaints, he was finally investigated and became deregistered to practice.

versus

A Known Lyme Doctor

A patient of a known Lyme doctor was laboratory-confirmed to have hypothyroidism and was under treatment.

Nevertheless, an endocrinologist complained to Australian Health Practitioner Regulation Agency (AHPRA) claiming a misdiagnosis of hypothyroidism.

The Lyme doctor's license was then suspended by the AHPRA.

The patient was re-tested and again the laboratory tests showed hypothyroidism. The Lyme doctor continues to have a suspended license.

50

© Copyright 2018. Global Network on Institutional Discrimination and
Ad Hoc Committee for Health Equity in ICD11 Borreliosis Codes. All Rights Reserved

VI.1.5. Bafflement and Restrictions in Ireland

SR Michel Forst, "The attacks take place against a backdrop in which business enterprises already have significant influence over States and ensure that regulations, policies and investment agreements are framed in a way that promotes the profitability of their business, often to the detriment of human rights."
—October 2017 to UN General Assembly

Dr. Jack Lambert is a member of the IDSA and is based in Dublin, Ireland [90]. He is consultant in infectious diseases (ID) at the Mater Hospital and Rotunda Maternity Hospital in Dublin, Professor of Medicine at the University College Dublin School of Medicine in Dublin, and Director of the National Isolation Unit for highly infectious diseases in Ireland. He has book chapters in 10 infectious diseases and other publications, and his CV includes over 120 publications in peer reviewed journals.

According to Lambert, the IDSA has provided him with the accurate and up-to-date knowledge on other severe infectious diseases, such as HIV , Hepatitis and Tuberculosis. However, this has not been the case with LB. His inspection of their documents on Lyme and co-infections (coinfections are other tick-borne pathogens that commonly accompany Borreliosis) show a very selective choice of studies, and not a comprehensive view of the subject.

Lambert notes that when it comes to Lyme and co-infections such as *Anaplasma*, *Babesia* and *Bartonella*, there is just a very limited or "censored" kind of opinion.

This puzzles Lambert, a veteran with experience treating patients with HIV, who often develop multiple debilitating coinfections. According to Lambert, ID specialists didn't have an antibody test for HIV until 1984 and they couldn't culture the virus until 1987. Nevertheless, ID specialists performed evaluations of gay men in New York in the 1980s and knew they were immuno-compromised and that they were infected with all these opportunistic infections.

The specialists knew there had to be something they missed and kept looking until it was found. It took a lot of hard work, science, resources and thinking 'outside of the box' to come up with the right diagnostics tests and later with medication which has changed the course of history with regards to HIV and AIDS.

During the early days of the AIDS crisis, when Lambert and the ID specialists he knew 'saw that something was wrong with a patient, they stood up for them'.

Lambert has seen many different infections in immuno-compromised hosts, like HIV, Hepatitis C, those immunocompromised by cancer treatment and transplant recipients. Many of the textbooks describing these

© Copyright 2018. Global Network on Institutional Discrimination and
Ad Hoc Committee for Health Equity in ICD11 Borreliosis Codes. All Rights Reserved

infections were written by his former mentors and bosses, some of whom were nominees for the Nobel prize in Medicine.

In the last couple of years, it has become very clear to Lambert that there are many similarities between HIV, Hepatitis C, transplant medicine and the many complications that patients with Lyme and co-infections live with.

He observes these infections can be just as damaging and debilitating as HIV and Hepatitis used to be before there were medicines to treat these conditions.

Lambert says that ID specialists have put energy and initiative into the evaluation, understanding and ultimately optimal treatment for Syphilis, Tuberculosis, HIV/AIDS and Hepatitis, among other diseases.

Why this is not done for Lyme and coinfections, which are affecting literally millions of people worldwide in a tragic way, is a mystery to Lambert.

Lambert is the only known ID consultant in Ireland who follows the ILADS Lyme Guidelines. ILADS clinical guidelines meet the 2011 IOM standards. Lambert has a large cohort of patients who had been misdiagnosed with other illnesses —including Myalgic Encephalopathy/Chronic Fatigue Syndrome (ME/CFS), Amyotrophic Lateral Sclerosis (ALS) and Multiple Sclerosis (MS) —and who are responding favorably to LB treatment.

Dutch Lyme advocate Fred Verdult is also living with HIV.

His ID doctors, who were so compassionate in their care of his HIV status, underwent significant behavior change when he got a persistent and complicated LB infection.

These previously compassionate professionals trivialized his experience. Their wrongful trust in the government recommended serology tests delayed diagnosis and treatment for two and one-half years.

They were unwilling to cooperate with an ID doctor with an open mind about Lyme, so Fred had to resolve difficult interaction issues between his HIV and Lyme treatments by himself.

According to Fred, this unprofessional response was a shock, a betrayal of trust and it had a very negative impact on his physical and mental health.

In Ireland, the demands for LB treatment have increased over the last three years. The laboratory tests submitted by Lambert for LB often included co-infections such as *Babesia*, *Anaplasma* and *Chlamydia pneumoniae*.

After he gave presentations on LB to a civil society organization and his knowledge and views were aired as a Lyme commentary in Ireland, Lambert was given certain restrictions. He can no longer test for co-infections and can only have LB tests done if he sends the samples out to the national virus reference laboratory.

© Copyright 2018. Global Network on Institutional Discrimination and
Ad Hoc Committee for Health Equity in ICD11 Borreliosis Codes. All Rights Reserved

Lambert has never seen obstruction of this sort for any of the other infectious diseases he treats patients for. Lambert was told they want to save money. Nevertheless, all his other colleagues order these tests; only he is restricted from making these orders.

Lambert is also restricted by how he can serve the public suffering from LB and coinfections. Lambert can still see established LB patients that came to his public clinic. However, new LB patients must see him privately and pay accordingly for service.

Altogether these restrictions create obstruction to diagnosis and care for those unable to pay for private clinical services.

These restrictions promote human rights violations and do not conform with the requirement for affordability under the Availability, Accessibility, Acceptability, Quality health rights endorsed by the Government of Ireland.

> "ACCESSIBILITY:
>
> Health facilities, goods, and services have to be accessible
>
> —physically accessible, affordable, and accessible information—
>
> to everyone within the jurisdiction of the State party without discrimination."
>
> —WHO principles

VII.   The Role of Financial Competition

VII.1. Sin Hang Lee

"The medical profession has been transformed into a "healthcare industry". In this world of free market economy, the healthcare providers in the pain management business may arguably have the rights to create public need for their services, just like Apple creating demand for its iPhone.

I cannot challenge a private group for conducting their normal business, but I can bring litigation against a competitor for anti-competitive activity..."
—Dr. Sin Hang Lee [90]

Sin Hang Lee, MD graduated from Wuhan Medical College in China. After a residency-fellowship at Cornell-New York Hospital and Memorial Hospital for Cancer, Dr. Lee was certified by the American Board of Pathology and obtained the F.R.C.P.(C) degree in 1966. He was on the faculty of McGill University, then Yale University from 1968-2004 while practicing hospital-based pathology. He has over 70 publications from a career that has spanned nearly six decades. Lee is currently the director of Milford Molecular Diagnostics, Milford, Connecticut. Lee has developed and published routine Sanger sequencing-based

© Copyright 2018. Global Network on Institutional Discrimination and
Ad Hoc Committee for Health Equity in ICD11 Borreliosis Codes. All Rights Reserved

diagnostic methods for HPV, *Neisseria gonorrhoeae*, *Chlamydia trachomatis*, Lyme disease borreliae and *BRCA*1/2 mutations implementable in community hospital laboratories.

Four months prior to the Texas suit filed by a group of Lyme patients, Lee initiated legal action against the CDC [13]. Lee alleges the "CDC implemented an anti-competitive campaign to stifle the use and availability of his DNA-based direct test to diagnose Lyme disease".

At the age of 85, Lee has unique and very informed perspective on the developments of the policies and politics of Lyme disease. He witnessed how Lyme arthritis was first described and reported in the world literature, and how patients have been diagnosed and treated in southern Connecticut over four decades.

Lyme borreliosis is a systemic bacterial infectious disease. Lee says, "According to the established principle in medical practice, all infectious diseases should be diagnosed by culture or detection of the nucleic acid of the causative agents in patient samples."

However, the technology of the Polymerase Chain Reaction (PCR) patent had already been purchased when the 1993 Nobel Prize for discovering the PCR technology was awarded and world-wide PCR patent rights did not expire until 2006.

> Lee "If Lyme disease were first described after the world-wide PCR patent expired, I am sure we would not have any diagnostic controversies today."

Prior to when the PCR technology was developed and became free of patent restrictions, heavy financial investments were made in other diagnostic technologies. With regards to LB, these investments were for patented antibody-based technologies for diagnostic tests and in developing vaccines related to Lyme disease.

According to the CDC, diagnostic antibody titers may not be measurable in Lyme disease patients until 4-6 weeks after infection. According to peer-reviewed published studies and US government Hazard Information Bulletins, the borrelial spirochetes have already invaded deep tissues within weeks of the infection and may not be eradicated as easily as in the early stage of the infection. Early diagnosis and timely treatment may cure most Lyme disease patients and these early interventions would reduce the need for pain management and other supportive therapies.

---

[13] Sin Hang Lee's documents for this legal case are available to the Special Rapporteurs and others, as requested.

© Copyright 2018. Global Network on Institutional Discrimination and
Ad Hoc Committee for Health Equity in ICD11 Borreliosis Codes. All Rights Reserved

In 2004, Lee was employed as a pathologist in Connecticut at Milford Hospital and began to develop routine molecular diagnostic methods using the PCR and DNA sequencing technologies [91]. Milford Hospital is based in Southern Connecticut, a Lyme endemic area. Therefore, after the worldwide PCR patent expired, Lee and his colleagues developed this technology for Lyme borreliosis to meet local health needs.

In 2008, the department of pathology staff and the doctors of the emergency room (ER) of Milford Hospital started a research project to test the blood samples of the patients who presented to the ER with possible Lyme borreliosis. The 'Milford' test was approved by the Connecticut State Department of Public Health under the Clinical Laboratory Improvement Amendments (CLIA) in 2009 for patient care.

> Lee and his colleagues at Milford Hospital developed the first nested PCR/DNA sequencing-based test to diagnose Lyme disease infections before the antibodies are measurable.

The technical paper on the test was published in April 2010 and the clinical paper in November 2010. It was the first direct blood test with DNA sequencing accuracy and a new DNA test that was useful for patient care.

> It was widely reported in the news media that this first PCR Lyme test with DNA sequencing accuracy can reduce the time between infection and treatment.

Lee was then fired from his job when a Yale medical group doctor became the new chairperson at Milford Hospital. This chairperson told the human resources director to fire Lee because 'Yale's serology-based Lyme diagnostic tests could not compete with Lee's nested PCR/DNA sequencing test to diagnose Lyme disease at early stage of infection'.

Lee then made formal legal complaint against Milford Hospital after the Hospital terminated his appointment and Milford Hospital rescinded their termination order. However, they stopped offering direct DNA testing for Lyme disease since the end of 2010; this occurred after the Yale medical group took over the management.

> It is common knowledge that the Yale medical group has focused on serology-based tests to diagnose Lyme disease at convalescent stage of the infection.

Yale's rheumatology department 'discovered' Lyme. Rather than trying to control and potentially eradicate the *Borrelia* infection, they instead offer supportive therapy. Prescribing pain killers and immunosuppressants for patients with 'post-

© Copyright 2018. Global Network on Institutional Discrimination and
Ad Hoc Committee for Health Equity in ICD11 Borreliosis Codes. All Rights Reserved

treatment Lyme disease syndrome' is a major business for the rheumatologists in Lyme disease-endemic areas.

Delaying diagnosis of Lyme disease infection until the patients are in convalescence is an effective way to maintain a high number of customers with this 'syndrome' for the pain management industry —this practice has been considered 'acceptable' for more than 30 years.

In contrast to Yale's serology-based tests, Lee's PCR technology can diagnose the infection before Lyme antibodies become measurable.

In 2014, without any explanation, the CDC negated a previously agreed project titled "An open label, multi-site evaluation to assess the accuracy of current diagnostic laboratory testing methods in comparison to nested PCR and DNA sequencing for the detection of Lyme disease and related borreliosis".

"This unfounded negation by the CDC of this planned project is the basis of my complaint and pending lawsuit against the CDC." [14] SH Lee

Lee says, "I must emphasize that my lawsuit is only against a few managers at the CDC. Over the years, I have known some very great and ethical CDC scientists. I have visited their labs and they have taught me a lot of molecular biology." Lee also refers to well documented situations:

- there are CDC officials who —in addition to their full salaries and benefits— have made personal financial gains through the private sector relationships they formed when securing patents
- these public servants have also been active in the preventing and stifling of the products, devices or methods set forth by their competitors

Unlike other wealthy democracies, the US government allows its officials to personally enrich themselves from patents while holding public office.

According to Professor of Microbiology Holly Ahern, the IDSA and the CDC have long coordinated their messaging around LB and the CDC does mislead the public [90].

Ahern cites the CDC website, "Before CDC will recommend new tests, their performance must be demonstrated to be equal to or better than the results of the existing procedure, and they must be FDA approved." She says, "The explicit use of the term "FDA approved" by the CDC is interesting, because currently there are no FDA approved tests for Lyme disease, and that includes the serological tests the CDC recommends".

---

[14] Monies won from the SH Lee law suit against the CDC will be used to establish affordable diagnostic centers for Lyme and other infections across the globe.

56

© Copyright 2018. Global Network on Institutional Discrimination and
Ad Hoc Committee for Health Equity in ICD11 Borreliosis Codes. All Rights Reserved

The CDC is different from the private sector because the CDC employees are government officials and public servants.

Their salaries are paid by tax money and their job is to protect the public health and well-being ... this includes any pain and suffering caused by unnecessarily delayed diagnosis and treatment of disease.

The CDC is violating their own principle for diagnosis of bacterial infectious diseases and allowing some CDC officers to intentionally suppress development and discourage the use of scientifically established direct DNA tests for reliable diagnosis of Lyme disease infections.

> "These public servants who knowingly work against public interest for a personal agenda and personal gain should be held accountable."
>
> SH Lee

VII.2. France

Similar situations exist in Europe. In France in February 2017, a wheelchair-bound patient long diagnosed with neurodegenerative illness was 'cured' by Prof. Christian Perronne after three months of antimicrobial treatment and began to ski again.

This patient had received a negative Lyme serology test similar to those promoted by the CDC, the IDSA and Yale. Before her LB treatment, she sent her blood to a veterinary lab. She had to give the name of a dog to have her blood tested by PCR. The PCR was positive for *Borrelia*. She has since lodged a complaint at the penal court for aggravated deceit.

In 2016, a consortium of 150 (and now 300) patients took legal actions in the civil court system against a Lyme serology manufacturer for the inaccuracy of their tests. French judges are now asking manufacturers to provide arguments to prove that their tests are valid. This will be challenging given all the studies that show the unreliability of such tests. The manufacturers told the judges they could not provide this information and were then fined by the courts for stalling the process.

Three legal actions have been taken in 2017 and 2018. The third complaint was lodged in criminal court by 59 patients in February 2018 —it is for aggravated deceit. The patients denounce the possible collusion between some health authorities, such as the French National Agency for Medicines and Health Products Safety (ANSM) the French National Reference Center for Borrelia (in Strasbourg) and the companies making the diagnostic tests for LB.

57

© Copyright 2018. Global Network on Institutional Discrimination and
Ad Hoc Committee for Health Equity in ICD11 Borreliosis Codes. All Rights Reserved

They denounce possible COIs for the Strasbourg-based reference center and denounce the fact that the reference center is in a situation of monopoly, acting as both judge and party. The center:

- self-evaluates its own serologic methods, developed with the manufacturers, and concludes than they are 100 percent reliable,
- evaluates test by other institutions that may compete with their own tests and conclude than they are not accurate (such as PCR).

Furthermore, when there is controversy over the reference center's tests, the French authorities ask the reference center to be the arbitrator of its own work and responsibilities —the authorities renewed the center's mandate in 2017.

VIII. Defenders or their Families are Denied Critically Needed Healthcare

There are human rights defenders for this patient group who also suffer from LB and/or LB and coinfections. Apart from sharing the same struggles for access to medical care with the patient group, there are cases whereby some defenders appear to be denied medical care for other health conditions.

Canadian Lawyer Jennifer Kravis is a well-known defender of LB patients' rights to diagnosis and treatment, particularly that of children infected and/or borne with the disease. She has provided testimony to the Parliament of Canada on these topics.

In 2016, using the 'standard' Canadian tests, Kravis' daughter was diagnosed with two tick-borne diseases; they were *bartonellosis* and Rocky Mountain Spotted Fever (RMSF). RMSF is widely recognized as very dangerous and can be fatal without treatment.

According to the Public Health Agency of Canada, "antibiotic therapy ... should be initiated at the onset of RMSF-like symptoms without waiting for laboratory confirmation of the diagnosis [92]. However, instead of treating her daughter, her general practitioner (GP) Dr. Joanne Fox, MD of Oakville, Ontario dropped her as a patient.

Kravis found another GP who requested a referral to an ID specialist to treat Kravis' daughter. In the Canadian system, this process routinely takes between 30 and 60 days for confirmation of the referral. Kravis and her GP have waited 18 months for a response and have repeated their requests.

58

© Copyright 2018. Global Network on Institutional Discrimination and
Ad Hoc Committee for Health Equity in ICD11 Borreliosis Codes. All Rights Reserved

According to the Public Health Agency of Canada, "63 laboratory-acquired infections have been reported as of date with 11 deaths" ... this is a 17.46 percent fatality rate for RMSF [93]. To date, Kravis' daughter has been denied treatment for RMSF and *bartonellosis* by her government's health system.

The next scenario demonstrates how any human rights defender for this patient group might be denied medical care.

American Jenna Luché-Thayer is a former Senior Advisor to the United Nations and US government on human rights, gender equality and government transparency and accountability.

For 17 years, Luché-Thayer was misdiagnosed with a number of diseases including MS and lupus. She was then properly diagnosed with LB and underwent treatment. Neurological symptoms returned two years later, and she experienced significant obstacles in securing necessary diagnostic tests. Luché-Thayer's neurological symptoms included intermittent loss of vision, the loss of the ability to hold items in her hands and many seizure symptoms. Among other incapacitations, she was unable to drive a car.

Over a period of three months, her GP made requests to her insurer for a Magnetic Resonance Imaging (MRI) scan which was denied twice 'as unnecessary'. 'Off record' conversations with sympathetic professionals at the insurance company indicated that it was common practice among insurers to deny 'non-mandatory' diagnostic tests for LB patients. One anonymously gave her guidance on how to secure the necessary tests.

In Canada, the manufacturers' insert for the ELISA serology test states 'a negative result shall not be used to rule out a case of Lyme disease'.

Yet the Canadian public health authorities are using the test explicitly against the manufacturers' instructions.

These State Actors also deny access to further testing with a Western Blot in the case of a negative ELISA.

Furthermore, the serology test details of the Western Blot banding patterns are withheld from medical practitioners and patients by the State Actors that control the National Microbiology Lab where all Western Blot testing is done. The banding patterns are a very important source of information to assist physicians in test interpretation.

This is private patient data which should be made available to patients and their health professionals.

Luché-Thayer then contacted a neurologist who had treated her for a head injury over 25 years earlier. According to this neurologist, who is a Professor Emeritus at Stanford University, the old injury should have been sufficient in and of itself to qualify for a magnetic resonance imaging (MRI) test. This neurologist sent his formal opinion to the insurer with a copy to her GP. The subsequent MRI, covered

59

© Copyright 2018. Global Network on Institutional Discrimination and
Ad Hoc Committee for Health Equity in ICD11 Borreliosis Codes. All Rights Reserved

by the insurer, showed a number of brain lesions —a not uncommon occurrence when LB has been long undiagnosed. Her symptoms resolved with antimicrobial treatment. It required almost five months to secure this test and treatment.

American Enrico Bruzzese became an internationally renowned human rights defender for his daughter Julia when her blessings by the Pope in 2015 made the news across many nations. Prior to the Papal blessing, Bruzzese had fought, and thoroughly documented, every form of discrimination and denial of medical care Julia experienced since becoming ill with Lyme and other co-infections.

Bruzzese has documented violations of Julia's rights to treatment options, including those enshrined in the Americans With Disabilities Act and terrifying acts of inhumane and degrading treatment. For example, Julia was carried into Columbia Presbyterian and straight into a bed. She was bed-bound there, and Columbia Presbyterian did not accommodate Julia's disability. When Julia needed to get out of the bed, her father Enrico had to be available to carry her, even for bathroom use.

The physical therapist would come to exercise Julia regularly. On this day, he literally pulled Julia out of bed, grabbed her tightly by the waist, pulling her left arm up around his shoulder and neck. As Julia's limp body hung off his shoulder and her right arm and legs dangled lifelessly, he attempted to make her walk. After roughly about five feet, he let Julia go and Julia's limp body fell to the floor. The therapist grabbed Julia's head just before it slammed to the concrete tiles. Julia's attending pediatrician believed this 'walk and drop exercise' would prove she was faking her physical disabilities.

Following the 2015 international media attention to Julia's case media, US media began to undertake in-depth stories about the circumstances surrounding Julia's tickborne diseases and mistreatment by the health care system. An interview with Enrico Bruzzese by Huib Kraaijeveld shows how, in addition to Julia's human rights violations by the US healthcare system, the CDC became personally involved in her case. The CDC official contributed intimidation, interference, defamation and misinformation to the challenges faced by the Bruzzeses.

Enrico Bruzzese: "Shortly after the Initial Adverse Determination by EmblemHealth (denial of coverage for treatment) and the airing of the I-Team investigative report by Pei-sze Cheng reference on Julia [15], we received an unexpected phone call from Christina Nelson, an epidemiologist with the Zoonotic Diseases Division at

---

[15] https://www.nbcnewyork.com/investigations/ Lyme-Disease-Insurance-Fight-Investigation-360476931.html

© Copyright 2018. Global Network on Institutional Discrimination and
Ad Hoc Committee for Health Equity in ICD11 Borreliosis Codes. All Rights Reserved

the CDC. Nelson's phone call was an attempt to discourage us from treating Julia for Lyme disease.

"She spoke very confidently and used fear tactics to deter me from following a Lyme disease path of treatment. On a second phone call months later, Dr. Nelson explained to me that all researchers and doctors who call themselves Lyme experts or Lyme researchers are "quacks" and if I continue on this path I could be leading my daughter down a dangerous road, even death. Both phone calls were recorded legally and are in my possession."

Following the blessing, and up until recently, Julia has tested positive for *Borrelia Burgdorferi*, [and coinfections] *Borrelia Miyamotoi, Tularemia, Bartonella* and *Babesia*. Julia also tested positive for neurological antibodies that have been commonly found in the elderly or strongly associated with Lyme disease."
Julia herself has become an internationally known human rights defender for access to medical care. Julia and her father continue to battle for coverage for her documented biological illness.

IX.   Respected Medical and Scientific Professionals Targeted

"Human rights defenders must be defined and accepted according to the rights they are defending and according to their own right to do so [11]*."*
—OHCR

According to a November 30, 2017 article in the 'Sciences et Avenir' journal, "Lyme disease could be a new health scandal in France" [94]. This article featured an interview with Alain Trautmann. Trautmann is an immunologist, the Research Director Emeritus at the Center for National Scientific Research (CNRS) and the Institut Cochin in Paris. He has degrees in neurobiology and immunology from Ecole Normale Supérieure and the University College London. He won the 2010 Silver Medal of the CNRS and works on cancer immunotherapy at the Institut Cochin.

Trautmann accuses the French Academy of Medicine and the French National Reference Center for LB of denying the reality of this disease and going against established scientific facts.

Trautmann is close to retirement, allowing him outspoken criticism. However, there are but few outspoken medical and scientific professionals who have escaped censure, threats to their license and livelihood, and limits to their medical and scientific practices.

61

© Copyright 2018. Global Network on Institutional Discrimination and
Ad Hoc Committee for Health Equity in ICD11 Borreliosis Codes. All Rights Reserved

IX.1. The Netherlands' Case and Quacks

In the Netherlands there are several institutions that attack doctors who are known to treat Lyme patients with complicated and persistent cases. These institutions include the National Health Inspection, the Medical Board and the Anti-Quack Association. Half of the doctors known to treat Lyme have been investigated and harassed by the authorities.

Dr. Geert Kingma [90], a private doctor practicing in Amsterdam, has over 30 years' experience and has treated approximately four thousand LB patients.

Kingma is not afraid to treat LB patients and publicly defends their right to treatment options that have met internationally accepted standards.

In 2012, the insurer Zilveren Kruis tried to reclaim 90 thousand euros (one hundred thousand dollars) in treatment costs from Kingma, with the claim that these 'treatments were not medically necessary'.

Kingma's lawyer responded and the insurers did not pursue their claim at that time.

In 2013, a pediatrician lodged a complaint against Kingma, alleging he had made a Lyme diagnosis based on an incorrect interpretation of lab results; therefore, the 16-year-old patient's IV treatment was incorrect.

This complaint led to an investigation by the National Health Inspection. When the investigators arrived at his clinic, they performed a comprehensive investigation as opposed to focusing on the case in the complaint. For example, the investigators

Sick Children are Taken from Caring Parents

In the Netherlands, an independent organization known as BVIKZ or Interest Group for Intensive Child Care, has undertaken an investigation into false claims of child neglect and abuse by the Dutch Child Protection Services [90]. As of March 29, 2017, BVIKZ had compiled and researched 168 individual cases. Over thirty percent of these cases are about children with Lyme disease.

Many of these children have the complicated and persistent forms of LB, or LB with other coinfections. The degree and duration of the illness often results in children missing school for extended periods of time.

BVIZK compiled a spreadsheet of what is being used as the basis for the allegations. For example, a couple of weeks of school absence (due to illness) is considered as damaging the 'cognitive well-being' of the child and thus framed as 'child abuse'.

According to BVIZK chairman Vera Hooglugt, these situations appear to be subjectively reinterpreted by Dutch Child Protection Services. Hooglugt says that they are only just seeing 'the tip of a much larger iceberg' of these false allegations.

© Copyright 2018. Global Network on Institutional Discrimination and
Ad Hoc Committee for Health Equity in ICD11 Borreliosis Codes. All Rights Reserved

searched every closet and room and the dates on relevant medical materials such as needles.

The investigators determined that the clinic needed to be closed until further notice for 'safety reasons' and that the doctor had one week to correct many problems including: paper towels instead of cloth towels; garbage bins had to be replaced; hand pumps for soap dispensers had to be replaced by electric 'touchless' soap dispensers; and all protocols had to be rewritten and so on. When asked for guidance regarding the protocols, the investigators did not provide specific requirements as to how protocols should be written.

Kingma made these corrections within one week. He then had a phone conversation with a high-ranking government official, who said he was surprised these corrections were already made as they had been planning to close the clinic for a longer time period.

During the week the clinic was closed, Kingma rewrote four binders of protocols and addressed all the investigators had required. These corrections cost approximately 12,000 dollars and a week of sleepless nights. Kingma had to demand they make a second visit immediately following the 'closed week' in order to receive the formal notice he could reopen his clinic.

The National Health Inspection came three more times that year to make further inspections. They specifically asked for ten files of Lyme patients; Kingma anonymized these files prior to handing them over to the inspectors. The inspectors later asked for another 10 files of patients and again Kingma anonymized these files prior to handing them over to the inspectors. The file review resulted in the end of the inspection and also demonstrated the original complaint was unfounded. However, this was never acknowledged in writing by the National Health Inspection.

The Dutch Anti-Quack Association plays an active role in discrediting LB patients and their human rights defenders. The following text has been excerpted from one of their public acts of stigmatization and defamation[16]. In December 2017, the former gynecologist and former Chairman of the Anti-Quack Association, Cees Renckens wrote,

"The most widespread fashion disease of the moment is undoubtedly chronic Lyme … Quacks flock to this syndrome [as do patients] desperately looking for doctors

---

[16] https://kloptdatwel.nl/2017/12/04/kwakzalvende-medici-verantwoordelijk-voor-rechterlijke-dwaling-over-chronische-lyme/ by Cees Renckens on December 4, 2017.

© Copyright 2018. Global Network on Institutional Discrimination and
Ad Hoc Committee for Health Equity in ICD11 Borreliosis Codes. All Rights Reserved

who accept that it is a physical illness. These doctors are only too happy to deal with the lamentable victims, especially young women.

In shock, I learned of a recent court decision in which health care insurer ... was forced by the judge in Arnhem to pay the bill that a patient with chronic Lyme had received from ... Quack Kingma. He [Kingma] has no contractual relationship with the insurer, but nevertheless the insurer was forced by the court to pay more than 7,000 euros [8,623 dollars].

[The case] Marleen Groeneveld was a psychiatric nurse when she suffered from unexplained mood swings and other vague complaints in 2011, which were only diagnosed as LB after a few years. Apparently, this diagnosis was not made by a neurologist who was consulted —he could not find any serological confirmation of the alleged Lyme— but the diagnosis was confirmed after sending her blood sample to a German laboratory.

In chronological order she was treated at the Spaarne Gasthuis in Hoofddorp, the Annadal Medical Center in Maastricht ... and Maasstad Hospital in Rotterdam ... by internal medicine specialist Dr. J.G. Den Hollander. In Rotterdam, the therapy consisted of a three-week intake with continuous administration of Ceftriaxone per infusion.

Her [Groeneveld's] family doctor ... referred her to quack Kingma in Amsterdam afterwards. [Kingma] gave her intravenous Ceftriaxone, an antibiotic, for twenty weeks after which the symptoms were reduced."

Renckens goes on to state, in his opinion, the many outrages this case presents; they include:

- the fact that the insurer had not challenged the diagnosis of chronic Lyme disease
- at least one, possibly even two medical specialists, believed that Groeneveld had a real and persistent infectious disease
- the acceptance that the Dutch treatment guidelines for LB are too restrictive and are acknowledgement they are based upon 2006 IDSA Lyme Guidelines that do not meet the 2011 IOM standards and have been withdrawn from the US federal website for CPGs
- the judge considered the German and American LB expertise provided to him when taking his decision
- the judge was hoodwinked into believing "these foreign guidelines —much different from the Dutch LB guidelines— were indeed 'evidence-based" when in fact the 'foreign guidelines' are ILADS Lyme guidelines that meet

© Copyright 2018. Global Network on Institutional Discrimination and
Ad Hoc Committee for Health Equity in ICD11 Borreliosis Codes. All Rights Reserved

internationally accepted standards for clinical practice guidelines set by the IOM in 2011
- the judge was again fooled into believing patient's remission can be attributed to the treatment by Kingma[17]

Renckens also recommended that the Disciplinary Board for Healthcare thoroughly question all the patient's doctors. This recommendation had a chilling effect. Den Hollander had been treating patients with complicated LB cases; following this December 2017 publication Den Hollander stopped treating such patients.

> BVIZK chairman Vera Hooglugt observed that "Apparently national [Dutch] Lyme policies dictate that after a few weeks of antibiotic treatment, the cause of the disease is suddenly a 'mental issue' regardless of the fact that these children are still as ill as before."

IX.2. Belgium

In Belgium, there are few doctors who treat LB patients who have complicated cases. Of those known to treat LB, 66 percent have been investigated, harassed and/or penalized by the Medical Board. The Medical Board is an organization run by medical doctors to monitor the practice of their colleagues.

One such GP works with many patients suffering from chronic illness and has successfully treated hundreds of LB patients from Belgium, the Netherlands and even the USA, UK and Australia [90]. She also testified on their behalf at disability benefits assessments.

In 2017, a dietary therapist and new patient, filed a complaint regarding 'communication about prices' to the Medical Board against this doctor. This complaint resulted in the Medical Board visiting the doctor's practice and the Medical Board holding a hearing on the case.

During the hearing, the doctor showed proof her client had been informed of and consented to those prices set by the doctor. However, the price of one diagnostic test, done by a laboratory that does its own pricing and invoicing independent of the Doctor, was not provided to the patient.

In this case, the Medical Board determined the situation allowed them to question all of the doctor's practices including risks associated with IV treatments and the choice of diagnostic tests. The Medical Board stated that a doctor should always

---

[17] On March 1,2018, Dr. Kingma reported to Huib Kraaijeveld that Marleen Groeneveld had recovered sufficiently to return to work.

65

© Copyright 2018. Global Network on Institutional Discrimination and
Ad Hoc Committee for Health Equity in ICD11 Borreliosis Codes. All Rights Reserved

be present during IV treatments, apparently disregarding the fact that the accused *is a doctor* who presides over these therapies. In addition, by law, the Medical Board is required to send a report of the meeting to the doctor, but no report was received.

Three months later, a visit was suddenly announced by phone — Medical Board called at 10 am and said they would arrive at 11 am for an on-site inspection. The doctor responded by asking they reschedule as she had set obligations, but they insisted on their demands. The spouse of the doctor also spoke to the authorities; this situation was described as "obstruction" by the Medical Board.

The next action by the Medical Board was preceded by a three week notice of their intent to have an on-site visit. They visited the office and inspected every aspect of the structure; they looked at the front doors, the file administration, took pictures of the house and the garden, of every information brochure in the waiting room, the brand of her computer, the fee structure and so on. They briefly reviewed one single patient file.

During this office inspection, the doctor again requested the report of the first meeting with the Medical Board and was allowed to make a copy of the report. However, the doctor did not receive a report of the Health authorities' visit to her office.

In December 2017, the Medical Board demanded the doctor defend herself in a 'debate' against charges with 'possible breaches in medical codes of conduct' based upon Royal Decree No. 79 of November 10, 1967 concerning the Order of the Physicians. The doctor asked to postpone the debate due to personal reasons (her mother-in-law was in critical situation with a brain tumor and needed extra care).

The Medical Board denied her request and without her defense, convicted the Doctor of five charges: (1) commercializing health care, (2) not practicing medicine according to the latest science, (3) collusion, (4) a lack of practices regard the provision of correct and purposeful information/not communicating properly with patients and (5) a lack of quality of care.

The doctor has been threatened with a six-month suspension from practice. Such a suspension will result in the doctor's loss income and probable bankruptcy, loss of work and pay for the doctor's employees and approximately 2,000 patients losing access to the doctor's care.

> The doctor under investigation also provided dietary guidance and therapy.
>
> It may be coincidental that the dietary therapist who filed the original complaint has now established her business in a new medical practice in the same town.

66

© Copyright 2018. Global Network on Institutional Discrimination and
Ad Hoc Committee for Health Equity in ICD11 Borreliosis Codes. All Rights Reserved

IX.3. Switzerland

In Switzerland, there is no specialist title or training as a specialist in Lyme borreliosis. Nevertheless, a medical doctor who was treating an LB patient was accused of "treating without proper qualifications" in a lawsuit's representing disability insurance concerning her patient. The insurer's lawyer used the opinions of a professor of infectious diseases who works as an expert for the federal insurance of disability to defame and libel the treating doctor.

The Swiss national disability insurance pays their experts, such as this ID Professor, between nine to 12 thousand dollars per case. Such expert opinions are used by private and public insurers to provide or deny coverage.

The patient was suing the insurer for disability compensation of lost wages. This patient tested positive for LB and was showing objective improvement under antibiotic care. However, the expert for the federal insurance of disability —*even though he never saw the patient*— indicated the patient did not have LB.

In the court case of this patient, the judge very quickly decided in favor of the insurance denial for disability coverage.

IX.4. Canada

Dr. Ernie Murakami was educated at the University of British Columbia (UBC) where he obtained his Bachelors in Immunology & Bacteriology, and continued on to achieve his MD. He has been honored and recognized for his efforts to further the education of fellow colleagues through the UBC, giving him the status of Clinical Associate Professor Emeritus. Dr. Murakami is the founder of the Dr. E. Murakami Centre for Lyme Research, Education and Assistance and has made it his life's work to further educate and treat Lyme in Canada.

After decades of providing unquestioned quality medical service Murakami was forced into retirement for treating patients suffering from persistent and complicated LB and other coinfections [95]. Murakami has shared how a

In Canada, patients face State sponsored health system obstruction to LB serology tests and clinical LB diagnosis.

Family doctors and GPs often say they are unfamiliar as to how to recognize clinical signs and symptoms and are therefore unable to perform a clinical assessment. Patients with clinical LB symptoms or related TBDs are routinely told by their GPs that the GP is "not allowed" to order LB serology test.

Then, when the GP tries to refer that patient to an ID specialist, the referral is denied on the basis that the patient does not have positive Lyme serology.

© Copyright 2018. Global Network on Institutional Discrimination and
Ad Hoc Committee for Health Equity in ICD11 Borreliosis Codes. All Rights Reserved

College of Physicians and Surgeons of British Columbia (BC) literally called him a 'zealot' from the beginning of their investigation. He was in his 70s when forced into retirement and is in his late 80s now and still actively educating on LB. Murakami was a general practitioner in Hope, BC, for decades.

Murakami's retirement resulted in hundreds of patients leaving BC to seek treatment in California, Washington, New York and Europe. This is because when Murakami retired there was no BC doctor to take over his practice.

Murakami became interested in LB decades ago after recognizing similarities between LB and long-term effects of syphilis. According to Murakami, many of his patients had been ill for a long time; they had been misdiagnosed or diagnosed with LB but had insufficient treatment. Murakami said, "I've helped a lot of people, saved their lives. I've taken a lot of people who are extremely ill and made them better, and yet they were investigating me."

On December 29, 2017, following the submission of the Antitrust Lawsuit against the IDSA, the Canadian federal public health authorities also removed direct links to the 2006 IDSA Lyme Guidelines.

However, these State Actors continue to promote the opinions of the 2006 IDSA Lyme Guidelines throughout Canada.

Murakami has noted that some doctors believe 30 days of treatment is all you need to cure this infection. According to Murakami, there is a growing group of doctors that have found many cases require longer periods of treatment.

Murakami's care resulted in 21 people leaving their wheelchairs. He also restored the health of a nurse who had been so mentally and physically incapacitated she could not be left alone. This nurse had seen 30 doctors before she came to him. A few months after her treatment with Murakami she was able to conceive and have a healthy baby.

In June 2017, Dr. Ben Boucher testified to the Special Rapporteur for Health and Human Rights regarding the human rights violations experienced by LB patients and their practitioners. Boucher is one of the many Canadian physicians who was policed out of business.

From 1979 until 2013, Dr. Boucher worked in primary health care in rural Cape Breton. For 34 years he served this community uninterrupted. From 2006 to 2013, in addition to his normal practice, he treated over 200 patients from across Canada for tick-borne diseases and coinfections including Lyme.

Dr. Boucher provided this service because many patients were unable to get a clinical diagnosis and treatment in their own communities. His practice came to the attention of the health authorities and although Lyme borreliosis is a clinical

68

© Copyright 2018. Global Network on Institutional Discrimination and
Ad Hoc Committee for Health Equity in ICD11 Borreliosis Codes. All Rights Reserved

diagnosis, he was forced to close his doors because unreliable diagnostic tests failed to confirm some of the infections.

IX.5. France

Christian Perronne, MD, PhD, Internal medicine, is highly qualified and a recognized expert in medicine and infectious diseases [90]. His extensive list of credentials includes:

- Professor of Infectious and Tropical Diseases at the Faculty of Medicine Paris-Ile de France-Ouest, University of Versailles-St Quentin en Yvelines (UVSQ), Paris-Saclay, France.
- Chief of the Department of Medicine at the Raymond Poincaré University Hospital in Garches and a member of the research unit for biostatistics biomathematics pharmacoepidemiology and infectious diseases.
- Vice-President of the Fédération française contre les maladies vectorielles à tiques (FFMVT, French federation against tick-borne diseases), and President of the scientific committee of the FFMVT.
- He was vice-chairman of the National Reference Centre on Tuberculosis and Mycobacteria at the Pasteur Institute in Paris until 1998
- Past-President of the French College of Professors of Infectious and Tropical Diseases (CMIT)
- Co-founder and past-President of the French Federation of Infectiology (FFI).
- President of the French National Technical Advisory Group of Experts on Immunisation (CTV)
- Chairman at the French Drug Agency (ANSM, ex-Afssaps), of the working group making national evidence-based guidelines for the antibiotic treatment of respiratory tract infections.
- Principal investigator of several major clinical trials on HIV, mycobacteria and viral hepatitis, for the Agence Nationale de Recherches sur le SIDA (ANRS, French agency for research on HIV and viral hepatitis).
- President of the Communicable diseases section at the Conseil Supérieur d'Hygiène Publique de France and then of the Communicable diseases commission at the High Council for Public Health (HCSP), making recommendations for the public health and vaccination policies until March 2016.
- Member of the scientific committee of the French Institute of Research in Microbiology and Infectious Diseases (IMMI, Inserm) until January 2013
- President of the National Council of Universities (CNU), subsection Infectious and Tropical Diseases.
- Member and co-chair of the European Advisory Group of Experts on Immunization (ETAGE) at WHO.
- Author or co-author of more than 300 scientific publications.

© Copyright 2018. Global Network on Institutional Discrimination and
Ad Hoc Committee for Health Equity in ICD11 Borreliosis Codes. All Rights Reserved

Lyme in the French media

Before 2015, some French journalists, including Chantal Perrin, Bernard and Benjamin Nicolas, Gwendoline dos Santos and Isabelle Léouffre, had written excellent reports concerning the persistence, complications and care and diagnosis issues regarding Lyme.

Then, in July 2016, an article written by Emmanuelle Anizon, Lyme Disease, this Epidemic that is Hidden from You! The 100 Physicians Raise the Alarm, captured the cover page of the popular weekly magazine L'Obs.

The article highlighted the '100 physician appeal' that was spearheaded by Prof. Perronne, Dr. Raouf Ghozzi and Dr. Thierry Medynski.

The appeal made strong and concise requests for the political and medical changes needed to address LB and other tick-borne diseases.

Since the L'Obs cover page, French media coverage of the LB epidemic has remained strong.

Perronne has been taking care of chronic Lyme patients since 1994 and has followed thousands of them.

He participated in the first HCSP working group on the prevention of tick-borne diseases. In 2010, the first HCSP report was released; it focused on prevention public education campaign. Authorities did not implement these recommendations and said the information may adversely impact tourism.

In 2014, the second HCSP report on diagnostic methods and treatment options found the serologic tests for Lyme were inadequate and generally unreliable. According to Perronne, the report found that 20 out of 33 Elisa tests for *Borrelia*, marketed in France, were not reliable; four out of 13 Western blot tests were not reliable, and there was need for accurate diagnostic tools for coinfections.

Despite the documented unreliability of the government-recommended serologic tests for LB, the second report launched an aggressive set of actions including persecutions against practitioners, pharmacists and laboratories that utilized more reliable serology technologies and therapies other than those described in the 2014 HCSP report.

The National Reference Center, located in Strasbourg, submitted complaints against laboratories, pharmacists and medical practitioners.

Pharmacist Bernard Christophe, who made a successful blend of herbs for phytotherapy, unexpectedly died of a heart-attack three days before his appeal —there had never been one patient complaint against him. Nor had there been patient complaints against any of the other medical professionals who lost their licenses and livelihoods.

70

© Copyright 2018. Global Network on Institutional Discrimination and
Ad Hoc Committee for Health Equity in ICD11 Borreliosis Codes. All Rights Reserved

Perronne reported that in September 2016, the health authorities, Minister of Health, Director General of Health, High Authority for Health (Haute Autorité de Santé, HAS) acknowledged that LB is a great public health problem and that diagnostic methods and treatment strategies should be revised.

Mrs. Marisol Touraine, the former Minister of Health, acknowledged publicly that many patients living with persistent and complicated LB cases are abandoned and rejected by the health system. She announced she was launching a National plan against Lyme disease and other tick-borne diseases. For the first time in France, public funds were given for Lyme borreliosis research and a research project of a national cohort of patients was planned.

A multi-disciplinary group of experts was established at HAS, including representatives of medical societies, physicians from several specialties, microbiologists, general practitioners, the National Reference Center for Borreliosis, patients, Lyme literate medical doctors and a PhD researcher from the federation FFMVT.

The goal is to find a consensus for diagnosis and treatment. If this is not possible, the federation asks for the possibility to have two standards of care accepted. Prof. Agnès Buzyn, who was president of the HAS and who facilitated the creation of this working group is the current Minister of Health.

Nevertheless, despite the consensus and collaboration among civil and State actors in France, there remain efforts to undermine any government commitments to address LB epidemic.

An October 26, 2017 article from the Academy of Medicine and Infectious and Tropical Diseases Commission 'denounced the deception about Lyme disease' and insisted the standard serology tests are reliable and high quality and that there was no need to provide anything but short-term antimicrobial therapy for systemic LB infection [96].

IX.6. Scandinavia

There are some distinct regional differences whereby State Actors and State entities violate the human rights of Lyme and relapsing fever borreliosis patients and their human rights defenders.

> Southern Sweden has one of Europe's highest rates of Lyme borreliosis that rivals the rate of the LB endemic US Northeast [97].

The Scandinavian region has been long admired for its human rights record and global activism in support of human rights. The Scandinavian region is well known

71

© Copyright 2018. Global Network on Institutional Discrimination and
Ad Hoc Committee for Health Equity in ICD11 Borreliosis Codes. All Rights Reserved

for its equitable access to healthcare through its tax based national healthcare systems. It is believed that if one resides in Scandinavia and pays taxes, one has access to care via the national healthcare systems.

However, with regards to the human rights of Lyme and relapsing fever borreliosis patients and their human rights defenders, the situation in Scandinavia is among the worst of all the wealthy and established democracies.

> Mats Lindström, a senior police official from Stockholm, spoke to journalist Pfeiffer about his wife Claudia.
>
> Claudia was bedridden for seven years before going to Dr. Sandström in February of 2016. "Within three months of receiving intravenous antibiotic treatment, she could get out of bed," he said.
>
> Lindström shared that Claudia is better, but not fully recovered ... however, she is out of wheelchair for the first time in seven years.
>
> During Claudia's long disability, the Swedish healthcare system only provided 'psychological services' and 'help with her daily living'.
>
> Claudia had to go to Germany to continue her treatment because the government removed Sandström's legal rights to treat this patient group.

IX.6.1. Sweden

The State Actors of Sweden aggressively punish and remove medical practitioners who treat persistent and complicated cases of Lyme borreliosis and co-infections. Sweden is a case in point. At this point in time, there are no medical practitioners who openly treat this suffering patient group.

According to a March 3, 2017 article on the Huffington Post by award-winning journalist Mary Beth Pfeiffer, 'patients are bereft over their loss of care from Dr. Kenneth Sandström' [98]. According to the article, the top doctor in Sweden for treatment of advanced LB was suspended from practicing medicine, leaving hundreds of patients without care in a country that has endemic LB.

Sandström has practiced medicine for over three decades and treated his first LB case about five years ago, when a registered nurse who had been diagnosed with multiple sclerosis asked him to treat her for possible Lyme borreliosis.

Sandström studied the scientific literature for several months and found that the LB can mimic MS, that many with LB are seronegative and that extended antimicrobials may reduce or halt the MS symptoms if they are caused by LB infection. He also underwent accredited training to ensure he implemented these therapies appropriately.

Sandström told the journalist "Twenty years of MS was gone." He also acknowledges that not all LB cases responded so well, however he has observed

© Copyright 2018. Global Network on Institutional Discrimination and
Ad Hoc Committee for Health Equity in ICD11 Borreliosis Codes. All Rights Reserved

overall, and at times, dramatic improvement from extended antimicrobial therapy.

Sandström said his license was suspended because he treated patients with longer courses of antibiotics than recommended by prevailing treatment guidelines for tick-borne diseases. Sandström had also been treating for co-infections, such as *Bartonella*.

Since having his license suspended, Sandström has become an active global defender of this patient group and has testified to the SR Dainius Pūras regarding the patients' human rights violations as well as the situation of their defenders.

When no Swedish doctor is allowed to treat complicated, persistent LB…

In one case, a young boy has twice tested positive for LB via lumbar puncture, the first time at the Stockholm South General Hospital (Sachska barnsjukhuset).

At age six, the young boy was given a short course of antibiotics to treat neuroborreliosis following his first positive test. Once this therapy ended the boy continued to show signs of neurological damage. Six months later, an MRI showed lesions (damage). His parents had to fight for one year to get follow up appointments. The doctors who are managing his case do not 'believe' in persistent LB infection.

At age seven, a second lumbar puncture again showed LB seropositive at Astrid Landgren's Hospital. The doctors decided not to treat with antibiotics because it was a 'false positive' and said, 'he is going to test positive for years.'   With no further investigation, these doctors gave the following diagnosis, 'post neuroborreliosis' diagnosis, attention deficit hyperactivity disorder (ADHD) and general speech impediment.

The child's psychologist wrote a letter to the families' social worker complaining the patient's mother was tired and overly concerned for her child and there was no reason for her worry. The social worker did not enter the complaint.

Stockholm South General Hospital admitted fault to sending the child home while still symptomatic and with no neurological follow-up scheduled. The hospital wants to use the case for staff training.

The child is now eight years old and is regularly out of school because of health complications. Signs of neurological damage continue to increase and now include significant word loss. The child continues to receive no medical care for LB infection.

© Copyright 2018. Global Network on Institutional Discrimination and
Ad Hoc Committee for Health Equity in ICD11 Borreliosis Codes. All Rights Reserved

IX.6.2. Norway

On September 2, 2013, the Norwegian Board of Health, a State Actor, revoked the medical authorization of Dr. Rolf Luneng of the Norsk Borreliose Center [90]. The case against Luneng was based on several reports of concern from, among others, Preben Aavitsland, a longstanding infection control physician at the National Centre for Public Health and recently an independent epidemiologist.

The complaints focused on Luneng's use of extended antimicrobial therapies for LB and antimalarial drugs for Babesiosis. Babesiosis is a tick-borne pathogen that is similar to malaria and is treated with antimalarial drugs. Babesiosis frequently coinfects along with Lyme.

> **Celebrity Patient Defends Doctor**
>
> Lars Thorbjørn Monsen is a world-renowned Sámi-Norwegian adventurer and journalist famous for backpacking expeditions in wilderness across Northern Canada, regions of Alaska and many Scandinavian countries.
>
> Monsen is also living with LB and co-infections and his health improved under Luneng's care.
>
> Monsen has used his celebrity status to bring global attention to the need for doctors in Norway such as Luneng and to defend Luneng's reputation.

During the course their investigation into Luneng, the Norwegian Board of Health violated the agreements set forth in the Helsinki declaration [99]:

*"**Unproven Interventions in Clinical Practice**: In the treatment of an individual patient, where proven interventions do not exist, or other known interventions have been ineffective, the physician, after seeking expert advice, with informed consent from the patient or a legally authorized representative, may use an unproven intervention if in the physician's judgement it offers hope of saving life, re-establishing health or alleviating suffering.*

This intervention should subsequently be made the object of research, designed to evaluate its safety and efficacy. In all cases, new information must be recorded and, where appropriate, made publicly available."

> Published studies confirm the presence of Babesiosis in Scandinavia and in Norway in particular [100].

The Health authorities and the departments such as Tick Center and the Public Health Institute (Flaattsenteret and Folkehelseinstituttet and others respectively) refused Luneng's several requests to do a retrospective study on this group of patients that would document the results and tolerance to the treatment. The authorities were not interested in whether the doctors' patients' health improved, their only concern was if the doctor was following the guidelines or not. The

74

© Copyright 2018. Global Network on Institutional Discrimination and
Ad Hoc Committee for Health Equity in ICD11 Borreliosis Codes. All Rights Reserved

authorities did not accept that Luneng followed the ILADS Lyme guidelines, validated by internationally accepted standards, when treating patients with disseminated borreliosis stage II and III.

Luneng's references from international research and studies publications were set aside with the excuses that 'only Norwegian research and studies' were accepted as documentation —though there have been few Norwegian studies done to date on these subjects.

Luneng's patients ardently supported their doctor in this ordeal, and to this day, several hundreds of his patients acknowledge how his care improved their health. Since being stripped of his license, the doctor continues to try to help patients and all those who might have become LB and TBD patient in ways that do not require a medical license. For example, he has run for political office, using his campaign to speak out about this patient group and patient rights regarding access to care and treatment options are in the center of his political platform.

Aavitsland, the person who made complaints against Luneng, has a documented history of trivializing, dismissing and defaming the LB patient group and their human rights defenders. According to his blogs, 'patients and practitioners are being infected by LB from an internet epidemic'.

Silent Microbiologist Fired

After publishing the 2013 article 'A simple method for the detection of live *Borrelia* spirochetes in human blood using classical microscopy techniques' [102], Norwegian microbiology professor Morten Laane was invited to give a lecture at a 2014 scientific conference in Oslo [90].

Laane's University threatened to fire him should he speak at the conference. So, he literally did not speak but he did show his presentation.

Professor Laane was then fired, his laboratory was closed, the website of the scientific journal was hacked, and his published article disappeared ... but a vigilant patient saved the article.

Like others who defame and then take aggressive actions that imperil the livelihoods and licenses of these defenders, Aavitsland ignores the peer-reviewed publications regarding the unreliability of the serology tests, the persistence of complications from Lyme borreliosis and the presence of coinfections, and spends time and energy attacking and stigmatizing the patient group and their defenders.

However, the LB views of Aavitsland are losing credibility in Norway. On January 5, 2018, a Norwegian LB patient received a court ruling to compensate her 10 years after inadequate LB treatment [101].

© Copyright 2018. Global Network on Institutional Discrimination and
Ad Hoc Committee for Health Equity in ICD11 Borreliosis Codes. All Rights Reserved

According to the Norwegian district court, Torunn Seim should have received treatment for her many LB symptoms after a tick bite, despite her negative test results. It would take four painful years before she received antibiotics in 2011, and eventually became well after successful treatment at the Norwegian Borreliose Center, under then Director Dr. Rolf Luneng.

The District Court and Court of Appeals says that negative antibody tests cannot rule out a diagnosis of LB. Nevertheless, according to Tone Synnestvedt, representing a Norwegian LB patient association, "We are aware of many who have reasonable cause to suspect LB, but have been rejected by the health care system due to negative antibody tests."

Seim says "My wish is that people will hear how difficult it is with these tests, and how unreliable they are. The State does not want to accept ... that it is possible to have Lyme borreliosis without the tests giving positive results."

LB is a clinical diagnosis. The Court states that Seim should have been offered antibiotic treatment for LB infection when she had the multiple rashes known as Erythema Migrans, stated that she had been bitten by ticks and had typical disease LB symptoms.

To date, there have been no penalties against those doctors who refused to treat Seim.

IX.6.3. Denmark

The Lyme borreliosis response in Denmark appears to be riddled with conflicts of interests (COIs) and stifled by the looming financial crisis in the healthcare sector. According to the Sustainable Governance Indicators (SGI) - 2015 Denmark Report [103]:

> "The main principles of health care in Denmark are as follows: universal health care for all citizens, regardless of economic circumstances...
>
> ... Although Denmark spends a lot on health care, the Organization for Economic Co-operation and Development (OECD) considers its performance to be "subpar" ...
>
> ... In 2012, health spending in Denmark was 11 percent of GDP, well above the OECD average of 9.3 percent and 7th place among (34) OECD countries when it comes to spending...

© Copyright 2018. Global Network on Institutional Discrimination and
Ad Hoc Committee for Health Equity in ICD11 Borreliosis Codes. All Rights Reserved

... Health care is financed by a specific tax which is part of the overall tax rate and over which regions have no control. In the OECD Economic Survey in 2012, it was pointed out that there is "a lack of consistency in assignment of responsibilities across levels of governments, which generates waste through duplication, weak control over spending and lack of incentives to provide cost-effective services.

... A particular challenge for the future is how to manage and finance the need and demand for health care."

The government of Denmark's management of the LB epidemic makes use of the IDSA guidelines; the 2014 Danish LB guidelines specifically refer to the outdated IDSA 2006 LB guidelines. The government of Denmark will only acknowledge Lyme borreliosis infection that test positive on the unreliable ELISA serology tests.

These State Actors appear to prioritize the rationing of health care costs over universal health care for all citizens, regardless of economic circumstances. Evidence of these practices follow:

- The Health Authority has allowed its 2006, 2010 and 2014 clinical practice guidelines for LB to be contaminated by frankly unethical COIs and have done nothing to correct this situation.

- Klaus Hansen, an LB guidelines author is also one of the DAKO/OXOID test inventors (now owned by Thermo Fisher). Hansen admitted he earns royalty money on every sale of the DAKO/Oxoid *Borrelia* antibody test kit used for LB diagnostics prior to the 2006 guidelines —including those used in Denmark.

- The Hansen COI predates the 2006 LB guidelines. However, this COI was not disclosed on the LB guidelines until 2010 and the disclosure resulted from complaints, media attention and political pressure.

The nature of this COI should have resulted in Hansen's recusal from the authoring of governmental guidelines that promote his personal financial gains. The nature of this COI should have resulted in a comprehensive review of the entire LB Guidelines' content for accuracy and integrity.

Numerous sources state that Denmark is a low-corruption country. However, like many modern wealthy industrialized nations, Denmark's health costs are increasing, and while its government institutions and officials are considering new private sector modalities to address their health care needs, they are being courted by some of the most powerful corporate interests in the world such as insurance and pharmaceutical industries.

77

© Copyright 2018. Global Network on Institutional Discrimination and
Ad Hoc Committee for Health Equity in ICD11 Borreliosis Codes. All Rights Reserved

Although Danish government officials might not be directly benefiting from these industries, these officials are often relying upon medical professionals who may have well established financial arrangements with these industries and COIs that work against public health and patient care.

Dr. Peter C. Gøtzsche, Director of the Nordic Cochrane Centre in Copenhagen, has done significant research on the Global corruption of medical care by big Pharma. He has published, e.g. Deadly Medicines and Organized Crime and lectures globally on the topic [42]. Gøtzsche has stated that 20 percent or more of the medical doctors in Denmark have relationships with, work for, or benefit from Big Pharma.

These relationships may account for the increasingly questionable behaviors infiltrating the Danish health authorities and medical system. For example, in 2010 the Danish health authorities had Dr. Court Pedersen advise medical practitioners on how to treat LB. Pedersen receives financial support from Merck, Sharp and Dohme (MSD) Roche, GlaxoSmithKline (GSK), Boehringer Ingngheim, Swedish Orphan (or Sobi), Janssen-Cilag (Tibotec), Gilead, Abbott, Bristol-Myers Squibb (BMS), Pfizer, Schering- Plow and is a member of the Institute Council, Statens Seruminstitut [104].

The situation in Denmark is so repressive for the defenders and this patient group that there are *no doctors openly treating persistent and complicated LB cases.*

The situation is also repressive for debilitated LB patients who advocate on the behalf of this marginalized patient group.

The Danish government's aggressive promotion of their recommended serology tests included their support for the messages presented in the documentary 'Cheating or Borrelia' produced by their government TV2 station.

These messages included the defamation of the Danish LB patient group and laboratories and practitioners who diagnose and treat persistent LB and co-infections.

The Danish government ignored every formal complaint filed by the patients who were stigmatized and falsely presented in the documentary.

The State Serum Institute (SSI) appears to have colluded with TV2. SSI states that it has the following practice, "All test responses and analyzes remain confidential in relation to third parties and are returned only to eligible healthcare professionals who have submitted tests."

© Copyright 2018. Global Network on Institutional Discrimination and
Ad Hoc Committee for Health Equity in ICD11 Borreliosis Codes. All Rights Reserved

Yet SSI allowed a TV2 journalist direct access to the diagnostic test results. In the case of TV2, no written authorization by SSI was granted to Ketil Johansen to receive the test answers. Correspondence from Kåre Mølbak, the Director of SSI Infectious Disease Preparedness division to Aase Høg of Bagsværd states,

"The SSI was contacted by a journalist from TV2, Ketil Johansen, in the spring, after referring from Kåre Mølbak. Ketil asked if we would help to test some samples for *Borrelia* antibodies when they were making a program about *Borrelia*. We said yes. Ketil made himself the blood test for himself and eight of his colleagues, and the samples were delivered here on SSI. After analysis of the samples, the answers were sent directly to Ketil Johansen."

In later correspondence, SSI changed its explanation. In response from the Ministry of Health of 3, 11, 2017 SSI states, "In relation to the specific case, it is SSI's assessment that it is an experimental nature (a mini-project) of societal interest".

However, there is no evidence of the necessary approval for this mini-project.

It should be noted that Kåre Mølbak co-authored an article with Ram Dessau. As previously stated, Dessau is the point person for ESGBOR and has been a key spokesperson defending the legitimacy and reliability of the government-recommended serology tests for Lyme borreliosis over many years [105].

State Tells Disabled Patient to Stop Advocating

A Danish LB advocate, on disability support for LB and complications, was told by her municipal government she was not to do her LB advocacy work.

According to the law, everybody may work voluntarily for up to four hours a week under Danish disability support.

There are no rules regarding limits on 'non-paid work' responsibilities like laundry, cooking, watching children or elderly. However, one's volunteer work must not be similar to the professional 'work' that one could be paid for.

The municipal rehabilitation team were concerned that her voluntary LB advocacy would interfere with her returning to work in her own company. The team took this decision without speaking to the LB volunteer about the energy needed to do four 'unstructured hours' of advocacy work versus complex professional work done under deadlines and did not consider that working in her own company is far more challenging than doing voluntary LB work.

The advocate then requested to have two hours for her voluntary work on LB and received agreement.

Shortly after the documentary was aired, it was discovered that TV2 executives were earning nearly double that of the executives in private TV networks in Denmark.

© Copyright 2018. Global Network on Institutional Discrimination and
Ad Hoc Committee for Health Equity in ICD11 Borreliosis Codes. All Rights Reserved

The harms caused by these State Actors and State entities include inhumane and degrading treatment of Tabitha Nielsen, the young mother whose health was improving under LB treatment in spite of her diagnosis by Danish specialist of incurable and fatal motor neuron disease.

Dr. David Martz, an internal medicine specialist, hematologist and oncologist published how his case of LB was misdiagnosed Motor neuron disease, which responded to extended antimicrobial therapies [18]. Dr. Martz's case is published in journal Acta Neurologica Scandinavica [106]. Like David, Tabitha was seeing improvement in her health … until the TV2 documentary resulted in the interruption of the financial support for her medical care.

IX.7. USA

The USA has over 50 cases of unfair legal processes and convictions. The following examples highlight how those chosen for these spurious charges, harassment and unfair trials were, without exception, recognized as the defenders of the human rights of Lyme borreliosis patients.

IX.7.1. Dr. Kari W. Bovenzi

In 2013, the website of the New York State Senate, Senator Kathleen A. Marchione announced the 2013 honoring women in New York award for Dr. Kari W. Bovenzi [107]. The following is excerpted from the announcement of her award:

> The Texas Antitrust case filed against the IDSA details how, "as a result of their speaking out, from 1997 to 2000, more than 50 physicians in New York, New Jersey, Connecticut, Michigan, Oregon, Rhode Island and Texas were investigated, disciplined or had had their licenses removed.
>
> Many of these doctors were reported to their medical boards by the Insurance [companies]." [72]

"Kari Bovenzi, MD. is a pediatrician and owner of Genesis Pediatrics, and has dedicated her career to helping others … Always one to think of new ways to help, Dr. Bovenzi speaks out to help raise public awareness of the growing regional concern of Lyme Disease and has assisted many families doing personal battle with the challenges of Lyme Disease at her pediatric practice. A selfless volunteer, Dr. Bovenzi is very active in the community. She served as a volunteer with the Kid's Celebration Children's Ministry at Grace Fellowship and as a board member for Alpha Pregnancy Care Center and the Loudonville Christian School and served as the co-chair of Capital Region

---

[18] Also see Dr. David Martz's video regarding his misdiagnosis with ALS and then his diagnosis with LB and recovery. https://www.youtube.com/watch?time_continue=232&v=UY9FdULDV6M

© Copyright 2018. Global Network on Institutional Discrimination and
Ad Hoc Committee for Health Equity in ICD11 Borreliosis Codes. All Rights Reserved

Heart Gallery, an organization formed to assist older children and sibling groups who are waiting for adoption.

For all she has done for others, Dr. Bovenzi was a recipient of the Capital Region Leaders in Business Award and the Community Leading Women Award. She is also a Diplomat of the National Board of Medical Examiners, has received the American Academy of Pediatrics Residency Scholarship Award, the Dean's Award for Outstanding Research Endeavors and has been named to the Dean's List. She also held positions of Adjunct Professor at SUNY Albany, Physician at the Emma Willard School and as WGY Radio's Children's Wellness Doctor... Dr. Bovenzi's life and work of helping children and serving the greater Capital Region testify to her character, courage and commitment as an inspirational woman of distinction."

Dr. Bovenzi openly treats children with complicated and persistent cases of LB and co-infections. Shortly following this award, Bovenzi became one of the six doctors who treat chronic Lyme patients who were targeted by the state New York State (NYS) Office of Professional Medical Conduct (OPMC) for treating Lyme.

IX.7.2. Dr. Charles Ray Jones

The following was excerpted from an April 5, 2011 article from Yale Daily News [108],

"Over the past four decades, Jones has treated roughly 10,000 children with severe chronic Lyme disease. Parents from all over the world bring their children to Jones, and many said they consider him their final hope.

Jones has already been brought before the Medical Board twice, both times receiving fines of $10,000 for procedural violations, which he claims threatens his ability to practice. Jones claims the high fines he received were due to the controversial length of his treatments, rather than because they caused any harm to his patients through his violations.

Jones has never been sued for medical malpractice. "I'm not being disciplined, I'm being harassed," Jones told the News."

Jones' patients and their families said their lives would not be the same without Jones' long-term course of treatment. Many said they have seen their children misdiagnosed with arthritis, dyslexia, or even autism —a result, they said, of the medical community's denial that chronic Lyme disease exists.

© Copyright 2018. Global Network on Institutional Discrimination and
Ad Hoc Committee for Health Equity in ICD11 Borreliosis Codes. All Rights Reserved

Jones said he recalls one child, Timmy, a 6-year-old who came into his office with his mother, unable to speak or comprehend others. Timmy had been diagnosed by previous doctors with autism, but his mother believed it could be Lyme disease. Jones agreed.

"I remember he was sitting in my lap. He couldn't talk, but he made eye contact well, showing signs of intelligence," Jones said. "I looked him in the eye, I touched his cheeks and said, 'I hope that I have the key that can unlock your brain."

Timmy then wiggled out of Jones' lap and ran around the office, Jones said. Following a positive test for Lyme disease, Jones began treatment. After roughly five months of antibiotics —far more than the generally prescribed three to six weeks— Timmy saw Jones for a second time. "He came back four or five months later," Jones said. "He didn't run in the door, he walked in the door. He put my hands on his cheeks, he looked me in the eye, and said, 'Thank you for giving me the key to my brain.'"

The walls of Jones' office are covered in pictures, cards, and paintings —small pieces of gratitude from his patients. One card has a familiar Y [for Yale] with a bulldog over it. A current pre-med sophomore, who asked to remain anonymous because of the rift between Yale's medical professors and Jones, credits her place at Yale in part to Jones. Lyme disease had affected her processing and auditory abilities, but after five years with Jones, she graduated valedictorian of her high school.

"I'm immensely grateful for Dr. Jones, and the role he's had in my life," she told the News. "But I do feel like I shouldn't use my name because I've heard some of my professors speak against chronic Lyme and those who treat it."

IX.7.3. Dr. Joseph Burrascano

Dr. Burrascano has been an outspoken defendant of LB patients' human rights for decades. On August 5, 1993, he testified in a hearing before the Committee on Labor and Human Resources, United States Senate, One Hundred Third Congress, first session, on examining the adequacy of current diagnostic measures and research activities in the prevention and treatment of Lyme disease [109]. Burrascano's testimony included the following statements:

"If standardized protocols for diagnosis and treatment are to be developed, then they should be devised in conjunction with practicing physicians and

© Copyright 2018. Global Network on Institutional Discrimination and
Ad Hoc Committee for Health Equity in ICD11 Borreliosis Codes. All Rights Reserved

exclude the current inner circle of biased individuals, many of whom have their own private agendas.

Investigate and curtail the secret connection between insurance companies and those so-called Lyme experts who oppose long-term therapy yet who are being paid by these same companies to perpetuate and publicize this view.

There is in this country a core group of university-based Lyme disease researchers and physicians whose opinions carry a great deal of weight. Unfortunately, many of them act unscientifically and unethically. They adhere to outdated, self-serving views and attempt to personally discredit those whose opinions differ from their own. They exert strong, ethically questionable influence on medical journals, which enables them to publish and promote articles that are badly flawed.

They work with Government agencies to bias the agenda of consensus meetings and have worked to exclude from these meetings and scientific seminars those with alternate opinions. They behave this way for reasons of personal or professional gain and are involved in obvious conflicts of interest.

They feel that when the patient fails to respond to their treatment regimen, which is a common occurrence, it is not because the treatment has failed, but because they have developed a new illness, what they call the "post Lyme syndrome." They claim that this is not an infectious problem, but a rheumatologic or arthritic malady due to activation of the immune system. The fact is, this cannot be related to any consistent abnormality, but it can be related to a persistent infection.

As further proof, vaccinated animals now in the vaccine trials whose immune system has been activated by Lyme disease have never developed this post Lyme syndrome. Yet on the other hand, there is a great deal of scientific proof that persistent infection can exist in these patients because the one-month treatment did not eradicate the infection. Indeed, many chronically ill patients whom these physicians have dismissed have gone on to respond to, positively, and even recover, when additional antibiotics are given.

It is also interesting to me that these individuals who promote this so-called "post Lyme syndrome" as a form of arthritis depend on funding from arthritis groups and agencies to earn their livelihood. Some of them are known to have received large consulting fees from insurance companies to advise the

© Copyright 2018. Global Network on Institutional Discrimination and
Ad Hoc Committee for Health Equity in ICD11 Borreliosis Codes. All Rights Reserved

companies to curtail coverage for any additional therapy beyond the arbitrary 30-day course. And this is even though the insurance companies do not do this for other illnesses.

Unfortunately, Lyme patients are being denied such therapy for political reasons and/or because insurance companies refuse to pay for these longer treatments. Finally, long-term studies on patients who are undertreated or untreated demonstrated the occurrence of severe illness more than a decade later, reminiscent of the findings of the notorious Tuskegee Study.

And indeed, I have to confess that today I feel that I am taking a personal risk, a large one, because I am stating these views publicly, for fear that I may suffer some repercussions despite the fact that many hundreds of physicians and many thousands of patients all over the world agree with what I am saying here today."

In 2000, Burrascano was prosecuted for medical misconduct by the NY State OPMC. Significantly, these charges were not based on even a single patient complaint. By 2000, Burrascano had already treated more than 7,000 Lyme patients from around the world over the past 15 years.

The OPMC procedures against Burrascano showed their bias from the start. In a letter to a Lyme patient in explaining the procedures used by the NY OPMC, Dr. Marks, Executive Secretary of the OPMC wrote "Rarely, if ever, have the published guidelines indicated that anything more than two to three weeks of antibiotics are required to cure Lyme disease."

> SR Michel Forst notes that "Defenders working on governance issues, promoting transparency and accountability on the part of States, and combating corruption are among the most at risk groups of defenders ... subject to relentless harassment and multiple types of threats and attacks. These defenders reported governments' reluctance to protect them, due to the numerous political and economic interests at stake [110]."

However, Dr. Marks' opinions are contradicted by numerous research articles in peer-reviewed biomedical journals, indicating that many LB patients are not cured by two to three weeks of antibiotics, that some of those are cured after months or years of antibiotic treatment, and some are never cured. Marks also ignored the peer-reviewed studies that demonstrated some of the ways that LB can evade immune response and resist the effects of antibiotics.

The OPMC charges proved to be unfounded, but the harassment continued over a period of seven years. Burrascano finally chose to close his practice.

© Copyright 2018. Global Network on Institutional Discrimination and
Ad Hoc Committee for Health Equity in ICD11 Borreliosis Codes. All Rights Reserved

X. Conclusions

As noted by SR Dainius Pūras, health is among the most corrupt sectors in many countries and this corruption is driven by global causes as well as the weakening of institutional accountability and transparency.

He described the insidious nature of this corruption and how it undermines previously fair practices of medical ethics and social justice; even illegal acts become normalized.

This report has detailed some corruption driving official public health and medical policy regarding Lyme borreliosis.

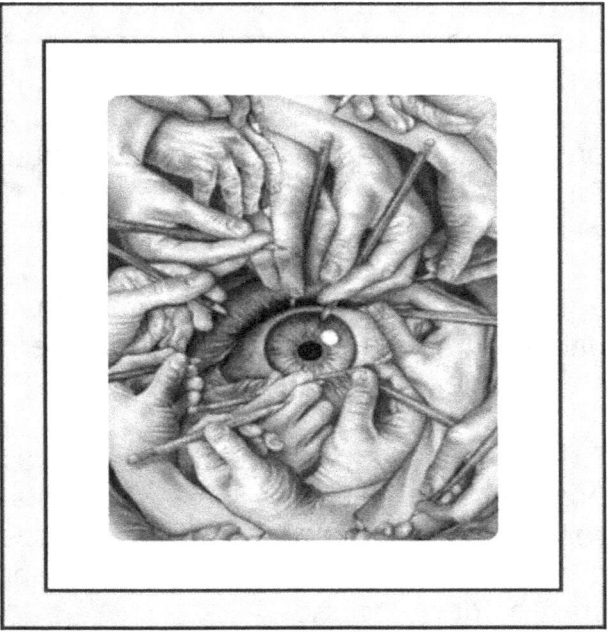

image source http://webneel.com

The propaganda promoted by these Actors is intent upon maintaining the status quo, that "Lyme is a mild illness, difficult to acquire, simple to diagnose and easy to treat".

The status quo maintenance is being implemented by a globally orchestrated propaganda campaign that is also protecting investments, perpetuating streams of research monies that result in few, if any benefits to patients, and certain medical and scientific technologies. One immediate financial incentive for maintaining the status quo is retaining and growing the market share for the increasing public demand of LB diagnostic tests. For example, patients who have received clinical LB diagnosis will pay for multiple unreliable serology diagnostic tests in the hopes of securing a positive test result.

This propaganda is also protecting financial interests such as insurers' increased profits and national health systems' maintenance of budgets by off-loading medical costs onto patients … and the pharmaceutical sector gaining hundreds of thousands of chronically ill persons who will require expensive symptom-modifying drugs for life.

© Copyright 2018. Global Network on Institutional Discrimination and
Ad Hoc Committee for Health Equity in ICD11 Borreliosis Codes. All Rights Reserved

There are many different actors involved in this corruption and many play an active role in distracting, confusing and misdirecting the public and well-intentioned medical and scientific professionals and government officials with propaganda broadcasted as medical and scientific information.

Experiences by the global advocacy movement to address Lyme borreliosis epidemic illustrates the undermining of historically sound government-stakeholder engagement processes.

> In his 2016 annual report to the UN General Assembly, Dainius Pūras expressed concern regarding the limited participation by civil society in many countries and insisted that, "States ensure that the decision-making processes that affect individuals' health and development are left open to such individuals" [111].

For example, in many wealthy and industrialized nations, citizens expect these engagements to adhere to the rule of law and be participatory, democratic, representative, accountable and transparent. However, in nation after nation, corruption and/or significant malfeasance and misconduct is evident during these stakeholder processes.

For example, the UK government's National Institute for Clinical Evidence (NICE) is currently implementing a participatory stakeholder process to develop their next Lyme clinical practice guidelines.

The NICE Lyme Guidelines Committee includes lay members and requested inputs from stakeholders including Lyme charities and patient support groups. A team collected data on all aspects of Lyme and generated more than 1000 pages of written reports documenting the evidence collected by the Committee. These included disease transmission mechanisms, diagnosis, testing and treatment and draft Lyme Guidelines for review by stakeholders.

> SR Michel Forst was "struck by the sophistication of the new techniques and forms of repression, especially via the media ... in several dozen countries, defamation campaigns in the written press or on the radio are routinely conducted by governments ... with a view to stigmatizing defenders" [110].

The stakeholder reviews were shared among patient-oriented groups and the NICE Lyme Guidelines Committee. The stakeholder reviews noted the demonstrated bias in the Guidelines and that well documented scientific evidence — including mother to fetus transmission, poor test sensitivity and reliability, evidence of persistence of disease, the failure of restricted treatment as

86

© Copyright 2018. Global Network on Institutional Discrimination and
Ad Hoc Committee for Health Equity in ICD11 Borreliosis Codes. All Rights Reserved

<table>
<tr><td>

Plans to interfere with CanLyme

Queens Lyme Disease Research Network (QLRN) is made up mainly of already funded and salaried government researchers, members of the AMMI and members of the IDSA.

QRLN held a conference in April of 2016 where:
- LB patients were referred to in negative terms.
- Dr. Muhammad Morshed of the British Columbia Centre for Disease Control *made a suggestion QLRN seek funding to build a website to lower the rankings of CanLyme on the internet.*

Morshed also contributed to the 2006 IDSA Lyme Guidelines.

</td></tr>
</table>

promoted by the IDSA— were ignored by the Committee. As of March 6, 2018, the Committee has ignored the inputs from all such reviews.

Lyme advocates question whether there was any genuine stakeholder process. This is, in part, due to one lay member of the NICE Lyme Guidelines Committee, representing a UK Lyme charity, who advertised many aspects of the draft Guidelines via social media almost 11 months prior to their public release [19].

This NICE Lyme Committee member claims to represent the LB patients' priorities but was promoting disability payments for LB patients *instead of* medical care and treatment options that have met internationally accepted standards. This Committee member is also on record stating that the UK's National Health Service (NHS) cannot afford these treatment options and cannot afford or manage to interpret more re liable diagnostic tests than those currently promoted.

Should those disabled by LB go on disability instead of receiving medical care, their disability support would be covered by the Department of Work and Pension (DWP) instead of NHS. Adoption of this recommendation by NICE would result in a cost savings for the NHS and an increase of costs for the DWP.

While this Committee member was promoting disability support rather than medical care, many thousands of UK citizens who were previously classified as disabled are being thrown off disability support. An August 2017 report by the UN Committee on the Rights of Persons with Disabilities concluded that the UK has failed to ensure the UN Convention on Disabled Peoples' Rights, to which it has been a signatory since 2007 and this discrimination is reflected in current UK policies and laws [112]. Furthermore, the UK government decided to 'incentivize' disabled people by trying to cut their desperately needed benefits [113].

---

[19] All statements made regarding this NICE Lyme Guidelines Committee member have supporting documentation provided by several UK Lyme patient support groups.

© Copyright 2018. Global Network on Institutional Discrimination and
Ad Hoc Committee for Health Equity in ICD11 Borreliosis Codes. All Rights Reserved

---

Twitter Attacks on Defenders of LB Patients by Government Grantee

Tara Moriarty is a PhD researcher at University of Toronto and a co-lead of a Canadian group called the Lyme Research Network (LRN).   LRN has been soliciting LB patients to participate in biobanks and patient registries. However, Canadian Lyme advocates and support groups across Canada unanimously declined LRN's request to participate in their research as they do not feel it is in patients' best interests.

Subsequently, Moriarty of LRN has been using twitter to discredit Lyme advocates; she has accused Sue Faber, co-founder of LymeHope of:
- "bullshitting people"
- "taking people for a ride"
- "exploiting people's fears" in a "sensationalistic" way

Moriarty also tweeted there is "no evidence of congenital transmission", this demonstrates a clear bias that repudiates many scientific publications. LRN is the only research network to have received any part of a four million dollar government grant currently available for LB research – a grant designed by the government of Canada to go to only one network. [114]

The promotion by this NICE Lyme Committee member for disability support *instead of medical care for LB patients* is particularly disturbing given the UK context regarding disability.

The preview of the NICE Lyme Guideline recommendations provided by this NICE Committee member indicated that the new guidelines would follow the opinion-based guidelines promoted by the IDSA; she also encouraged patient groups to accept the status quo ... meaning treatment options that meet internationally accepted standards would not be recognized or honored and, in many cases, positive tests results from unreliable serology tests would confirm the need for treatment.

As noted, many of the views of this Committee member were reflected in the NICE Lyme Guidelines draft that was publicly shared nearly 11 months later. Public comments by stakeholders who are pro-patient centered healthcare and represent non-IDSA views, and the many hundreds of peer-reviewed publications showing persistent infection and complications ignored by the IDSA, have also been ignored by the NICE Lyme Committee. Also noted, in violation of their own government regulations, the NICE Lyme Guidelines Committee has been actively promoting for use the draft version of the new Lyme guidelines to hospitals and other medical establishments.

Many UK Lyme advocates characterize the process as disingenuous, disrespectful, suppressing important scientific and medical knowledge, and politically and financially motivated by powers that have little interest in the health and welfare of LB patients and future LB patients[20].

---

[20] The views have been collected from numerous exchanges with representatives of multiple Lyme support groups

88

© Copyright 2018. Global Network on Institutional Discrimination and
Ad Hoc Committee for Health Equity in ICD11 Borreliosis Codes. All Rights Reserved

Dr. Perronne is Labeled a Terrorist

Dr. Perronne gave a plenary presentation at the National Academy of Medicine on September 21, 2016 in France. The balcony was full of journalists, Lyme patients and Lyme doctors and the Academicians sat in the main floor area.

Perronne's presentation demonstrated the poor reliability of the LB diagnostic tests, the persistence of *Borrelia*, the existence of co-infections and the lack of good studies to evaluate treatments. He also provided many published references to support his presentation.

A former professor of infectious diseases in Paris and former President of the Academy, Prof. Marc Gentilini (retired), shared his views regarding Perronne's presentation during the following question session.

Perronne remembers that Gentilini began his comments with, "I order you to retract immediately". Gentilini went on to say that Perronne had given "an irrational talk" and that he was a "terrorist".

Loud boos came from the balcony. Perronne stayed calm and gently but firmly responded to the charges by Gentilini. Loud applause followed Perronne's response. Gentilini's face then paled in color.

In a similar manner in 2017 in Canada, Canadian LB patients' participation and contributions were entirely and illegally erased from the Canadian government's final Lyme Guidelines product. To note, many of these contributions were made by highly qualified medical and scientific professionals.

The government of Denmark, including the government of Denmark's TV2 network, has made no apology or reparations for their disrespectful and degrading the mischaracterization of LB patients in their 'Cheating or Borrelia' documentary. The government of Denmark has casually dismissed the COIs surrounding the serology tests promoted by Klaus Hansen and the Danish Lyme guidelines.

As noted, the CDC, in flagrant violation of federal law, shows strong preferential treatment for the 2006 IDSA Lyme guidelines. Other US government institutions, responsible for ensuring the CDC act legally and ethically, have stood by silently despite multiple formal complaints over multiple years.

The NIH Office of Research Integrity has shown no action in response to multiple complaints over multiple years regarding the misuse of grant monies to stigmatize LB patients and their human rights defenders and the HHS Office of Civil Rights, an entity responsible for protecting vulnerable people from discrimination in health services and care, has misrepresented and misdirected complaints that provided comprehensive documentation of discrimination against this patient group.

89

© Copyright 2018. Global Network on Institutional Discrimination and
Ad Hoc Committee for Health Equity in ICD11 Borreliosis Codes. All Rights Reserved

In order to best understand the corruption surrounding Lyme borreliosis and co-infections it is necessary to note that there are other patient groups experiencing similar marginalization, stigmatization and human rights abuses. Furthermore, their human rights defenders are experiencing, to a similar degree, the human rights abuse of those protecting the Lyme and relapsing fever borreliosis patient population.

For example, ME and LB are 'emerging illnesses' that have been emerging for four decades. It is estimated that there are between 15 and 30 million persons worldwide suffering from Myalgic Encephalopathy (ME), also known as Chronic Fatigue Syndrome (CFS). The few doctors willing to openly treat ME patients are also routinely harassed, discredited and threatened in the same manner as our LB doctors and scientists.

The worldwide guidelines on ME are based on findings from the 2011 Lancet publication of the <u>Pacing, graded Activity, and Cognitive behavior therapy, a randomized Evaluation</u> or PACE trial. These ME guidelines have come under increasing international scientific and medical scrutiny.

The PACE study was funded by the UK government's Department of Work and Pension; the same agency responsible for supporting disabled LB patients.

The study compared 'standardized specialist medical care' (SMC) alone to SMC plus Adaptive Pacing Therapy, Cognitive Behavioral Therapy (CBT), or Graded Exercise Therapy (GET). The experimenters determined that the patients who received CBT and GET did better than other groups of ME.

ME Advocates Demonized

In 2014, ME advocates again initiated freedom of information (FOI) requests regarding the PACE data.

While these FOI requests were under consideration, Queen Mary University of London and the PACE researchers adopted a policy of demonizing ME patients who criticized the PACE trial by portraying them as 'unreasonable, obsessive, unstable, and dangerous malcontents.'

These findings have been very influential; they were used to formulate NICE's ME Guidelines for clinical practice and have been adopted by most nations including USA, the Netherlands, Canada, Scandinavian countries. Policies based on PACE are used to determine coverage by both government funded healthcare and private medical insurers. The draft ICD 11 codes for ME have been moved from neurological conditions to "disorders of consciousness".

Forty-two scientists and clinicians wrote an open letter to the Lancet criticizing the PACE study's authors violation of the Declaration of Helsinki, which mandates that prospective

© Copyright 2018. Global Network on Institutional Discrimination and
Ad Hoc Committee for Health Equity in ICD11 Borreliosis Codes. All Rights Reserved

participants be 'adequately informed' about researchers' "possible conflicts of interest" [115]. The letter states,

"The main [PACE] investigators have had financial and consulting relationships with disability insurance companies, advising them that rehabilitative therapies like those tested in PACE could help ME/CFS claimants get off benefits and back to work. They disclosed these insurance industry links in The Lancet but did not inform trial participants, contrary to their protocol commitment. This serious ethical breach raises concerns about whether the consent obtained from the 641 trial participants is legitimate."

More analysis by independent research groups indicate the PACE findings to be unduly biased and/or fraudulent. [116] The reanalysis of the raw data calls into question the research integrity of the PACE trials as a well as NICE's recent attempts to again 'formulate ME guidelines' based on PACE findings. This has led to hearings and debates in the Scottish Parliament [117]

These developments have contributed to ME advocates successful disruption of NICE's attempts to again base their ME Guidelines on the PACE trial. On 14th January 2018, Dr. Sarah Myhill made formal complaint regarding the PACE trial to Sir Terence Stephenson, the Chair of the General Medical Council. Myhill is spearheading efforts to have a Public Inquiry into the medical abuse of ME sufferers.

NICE, the same entity responsible for promoting PACE as a basis for ME treatment, is currently reformulating the Lyme Guidelines and they mirror the opinions found in the IDSA 2006 Lyme Guidelines.

ME patients, like Lyme and relapsing fever borreliosis patients, have witnessed a cohort of actors representing the State and private interests deliberately suppress the scientific and medical evidence showing these complex systemic illnesses are biological in nature and promote the fraud that these patients are basically ill-adjusted hypochondriacs undeserving of medical care.

Like Lyme and relapsing fever borreliosis patients, ME patients and their families bear the personal brunt of the medical costs and the degradation of inhumane treatment by the health care system.

Both patient groups have shared the disrespectful humiliation of pretense by government officials who employ gaslighting techniques while claiming to consider patient priorities when developing policies that have to date, undermined their health and the financial solvency of their families.

© Copyright 2018. Global Network on Institutional Discrimination and
Ad Hoc Committee for Health Equity in ICD11 Borreliosis Codes. All Rights Reserved

"An excellent example of the failure to comprehend the interface between the brain and body is the concept of so called "bodily distress syndrome," which is a very distressing concept. The term was never given any validity in any edition of the American Psychiatric Association Diagnostic and Statistical Manual (APA DSM) and was not even recognized as a condition needing further research. "Bodily distress syndrome" is basically a synonym for "Medically Unexplained Symptoms," a concept that is recognized to lack validity in the APA DSM-5.

It appears no psychiatrists and no psychiatric organizations have ever endorsed the bodily distress syndrome concept ... but significant financial interests seem to be indicated as the prime movers. Furthermore, there are now significant efforts to have "Bodily distress syndrome" overlap with the "Bodily distress disorder" presented in the WHO's ICD11 codes."

Robert C. Bransfield,
MD, DLFAPA Psychiatrist

Robert C. Bransfield [21]

ME patients, mostly children patients, have been forcibly removed from their homes, forcibly required to implement the PACE protocols and died as result.

In addition to the ME and Lyme and relapsing fever borreliosis patient groups, there are other patient groups with complex illnesses who are being systematically humiliated, degraded, stigmatized and denied adequate medical care.

In many cases, this pattern of corruption and fraud is accompanied by fabricated psychosomatic labels such as 'medically unexplained symptoms', 'bodily distress disorder' and 'bodily distress syndrome'.

These deceptive terms are now also being applied to an increasing number of patient groups that were previously recognized as having medical conditions and are currently being deliberately 'somaticized' away from medical care. These patient groups include persons with traumatic brain injury and females with extensive noncancerous growths and adhesions surrounding their reproductive organs who have 'symptoms lasting more than six months'.

---

[21] Robert C. Bransfield, MD, DLFAPA is in the private practice of psychiatry. He is an Associate Clinical Professor at Rutgers-RWJ School of Medicine and Past President of the New Jersey Psychiatric Association, the ILADS and the International Lyme and Associated Diseases Educational Foundation. Bransfield is board certified by the American Board of Psychiatry and Neurology and is a Distinguished Life Fellow of the American Psychiatric Association. He earned his medical degree from the George Washington University School of Medicine in Washington, DC and completed a residency in psychiatry at Sheppard and Enoch Pratt Hospital. Bransfield has an interest in healthcare policy and the association between infections, psychoimmunology and mental illness. He has authored a number of publications in peer-reviewed literature, other medical publications, and books; has presented at numerous medical conferences, both nationally and internationally, and has appeared on network and regional television and radio.

© Copyright 2018. Global Network on Institutional Discrimination and
Ad Hoc Committee for Health Equity in ICD11 Borreliosis Codes. All Rights Reserved

"The synonym of bodily distress syndrome, Medically Unexplained Symptoms, is not included in the APA DSM-5 because "no medical condition is totally explained or unexplained. Instead, knowledge is on a continuum and all conditions are partially explained to different degrees.

This label is impacted by the bias and level of knowledge of anyone calling it 'unexplained.' These symptoms are often unexamined rather than unexplained [45]."

Robert C. Bransfield,
MD, DLFAPA Psychiatrist

SR Dainius Pūras has emphasized the "normalization" of corruption in healthcare and noted how such practices undermine medical ethics, social justice, transparency and effective healthcare provision and promote or protect illegal acts.

The health sector corruption pandemic is creating increasing numbers of patient groups who routinely experience human rights abuses. This corruption is a threat to sustainable development goals, government transparency and accountability, and the promises made to protect human rights and no less than 11 international and/or regional human rights treaties and covenants.

This threat requires a comprehensive response by key institutions beyond those found in the healthcare system.

The following recommendations identify feasible priorities within this complex and compromised mesh of medical, scientific, legal, social, economic and governmental practices.

Solutions

1. Provide public funding to improve borreliosis diagnostic tests, which are currently unreliable. There should be a portion of this funding set aside for new innovators.

2. Until such tests are available, recognize and honor, support and accept the clinical diagnosis of Lyme borreliosis.

3. Create enabling environments for multiple innovative diagnostic tests to compete with those patents and reagents held by the CDC and other institutions holding outdated patents.

4. Change the laws so that government institutions and officials responsible for promoting scientific and medical innovations cannot be patent holders in the same arenas of competition.

93

© Copyright 2018. Global Network on Institutional Discrimination and
Ad Hoc Committee for Health Equity in ICD11 Borreliosis Codes. All Rights Reserved

5. Prioritize research on interhuman transmission such as congenital LB, possible sexual transmission and transmission via blood transfusions and organ donors.

6. Modernize the WHO's International Classification of Diseases (ICD) codes for Lyme borreliosis to reflect the complexity and seriousness of the disease.

7. Modernize the WHO's ICD codes for relapsing fever borreliosis.

8. Utilize the improved ICD codes to enhance the quality of borreliosis surveillance to:
   - inform public health policy
   - strengthen the 'One Health' synergy - to obtain optimal health of people, animals, and the environment
   - understand and prepare for the impact of climate change

9. Official recognition of complicated and persistent Lyme borreliosis is required

10. Official recognition of physical disability caused by Lyme borreliosis is required.

11. Require national health systems and private insurers to recognize and provide treatment coverage for complicated and persistent forms of Lyme borreliosis. Qualifying treatments would include those that meet (US) Institutional of Medicine's (IOM) 2011 internationally accepted standards for clinical practice guidelines.

12. Stop the persecution of doctors who utilize clinical diagnosis and treatments that meet IOM 2011 standards for clinical practice guidelines.

13. Penalize the slandering, libeling, stigmatizing and bullying of Lyme patients.

14. Make the differential diagnosis of Lyme borreliosis part of standard medical assessments in countries where the diseases have been identified.

    The lack of differential diagnosis is particularly problematic for certain groups – such as the elderly. For example, untreated Lyme borreliosis symptoms can mimic conditions associated with aging, e.g. arthritis, dementia and vision and hearing loss.

15. Honor patients' rights to choose among treatment options and require medical professionals to inform patients of these choices.

16. Increase public funding for patient-centered research to improve diagnosis and treatments for borreliosis, other tick-borne diseases and co-infections.

94

© Copyright 2018. Global Network on Institutional Discrimination and
Ad Hoc Committee for Health Equity in ICD11 Borreliosis Codes. All Rights Reserved

17. In many countries, children are among in the highest risk groups for Lyme borreliosis. Help these children reach their potential and fulfill their dreams by organizing collaboration among key institutions to protect the health and advancement of these children.

18. Require public schools and universities to develop plans to accommodate students living with complicated and persistent forms of Lyme borreliosis.

19. Require public institutions provide those living with Lyme and relapsing fever borreliosis (and co-infections) full access to their services.

20. Assist private businesses and corporations in developing employer strategies that retain employees who have debilitation or other limitations due to Lyme and relapsing fever borreliosis (and co-infections).

21. Require that all standing governmental committees for borreliosis research and policy have democratic, transparent and representative stakeholder inclusion of patients and caretakers.

Many governments now recognize that healthcare and disability costs are unsustainable and may undermine their national economies. Nevertheless, current practices regarding healthcare cost considerations are largely reduced to insurers' quarterly earnings and governments' annual budgets.

This short-term thinking is disastrous with regards to the unsustainable healthcare and disability costs from the expanding pandemic of undiagnosed, misdiagnosed, untreated and/or undertreated Lyme and relapsing fever borreliosis patients.

Affordable access to a variety of diagnostic tests and all treatment options that meet international standards will greatly reduce this projected burden. Furthermore, properly recognizing and addressing the Lyme and relapsing fever borreliosis pandemic will serve economic and humanitarian goals.

© Copyright 2018. Global Network on Institutional Discrimination and
Ad Hoc Committee for Health Equity in ICD11 Borreliosis Codes. All Rights Reserved

*"In the fullness of time,
the mainstream handling of Chronic Lyme disease
will be viewed as one of the most shameful episodes in the history of medicine
because elements of academic medicine, elements of government
and virtually the entire insurance industry
have colluded to deny a disease."*[22]

—Dr. Kenneth Liegner
Lyme patients' human rights defender for 40 years

[22] September 14, 2010 Letter from Kenneth B. Liegner, M.D., P.C. to Lonnie King, Trevonne Walford, Christine M. Coussens, Members of the IOM Committee Panel for "Lyme Disease & Other Tick-borne Diseases: State of the Science" Institute of Medicine of The National Academy of Sciences. Keck Center, 500 Fifth St. NW, Washington, DC 20001

© Copyright 2018. Global Network on Institutional Discrimination and
Ad Hoc Committee for Health Equity in ICD11 Borreliosis Codes. All Rights Reserved

References

[1]   http://www.ohchr.org/EN/NewsEvents/Pages/DisplayNews.aspx?NewsID=22283
&LangID=E

[2]   MacDonald AB, Benach JL, Burgdorfer W. Stillbirth following maternal Lyme
disease. N Y State J Med. 1987;11:615-616.

[3]   Macdonald AB. Human fetal borreliosis, toxemia of pregnancy, and fetal death.
Zentralblatt für Bakteriologie, Mikrobiologie und Hygiene. Series A: Medical
Microbiology, Infectious Diseases, Virology, Parasitology. 1986;263(1-2):189-
200. doi:10.1016/s0176-6724(86)80122-5. klinische Wochenschrift.
2000;111:933-40.

[4]   Markowitz LE, Steere AC, Benach JL, Slade JD, Broome CV. Lyme disease during
pregnancy. JAMA: The Journal of the American Medical Association.
1986;255(24):3394. doi:10.1001/jama.1986.03370240064038. PubMed

[5]   Schlesinger PA, Duray PH, Burke BA, Steere AC, Stillman MT. Maternal-fetal
transmission of the Lyme disease Spirochete, Borrelia burgdorferi. Annals of
Internal Medicine. 1985;103(1):67. doi:10.7326/0003-4819-103-1-67.

[6]   Silver RM, Yang L, Daynes RA, Branch WD, Salafia CM, Weis JJ. Fetal outcome
in Murine Lyme disease. Infection and Immunity. 1995;63(1):66-72.

[7]   Strobino BA, Williams CL, Abid S, Ghalson R, Spierling P. Lyme disease and
pregnancy outcome: A prospective s of two thousand prenatal patients.
American Journal of Obstetrics and Gynecology. 1993;169(2):367-374.
doi:10.1016/0002-9378(93)90088-z.

[8]   Weber K, Bratzke H-J, Neubert U, Wilske B, Duray PH. Borrelia burgdorferi in a
newborn despite oral penicillin for Lyme borreliosis during pregnancy. The
Pediatric Infectious Disease Journal. 1988;7(4):286-288. doi:10.1097/00006454-
198804000-00010.

[9]   LaPenta, Jose. Investigative Dermatology and Venereology Research (Journal)
January 12, 2.018. https://doi.org/10.15436/2381-0858.18.1769
https://www.ommegaonline.org/article-details/UNDERSTANDING-THE-LYME-
DISEASE,-CLASSIFICATION-AND-CODES./1769

[10]   Luché-Thayer J, Ahern H, DellaSala D, Franklin S, Gilbert L, Horowitz R,
Liegner K, McManus M, Meseko C, Miklossy J, Rudenko N, Stuckelberger A.
Updating ICD11 Borreliosis Diagnostic Codes: Edition One, March 29, 2017.
Contributing researchers: Joseph Beaton, John Blakely, Phyllis Freeman, Kunal
Garg, Huib Kraaijeveld, Vett Lloyd, Leena Meriläinen. Cees Hamelink, Advisor
Jeff Levy, editorial support Angelica Johannson, organizational support. ISBN-
10: 1978091796 ISBN-13: 978-1978091795 CreateSpace Independent Publishing
Platform October 7, 2017.

[11]   http://www.ohchr.org/EN/Issues/SRHRDefenders/Pages/Defender.aspx

© Copyright 2018. Global Network on Institutional Discrimination and
Ad Hoc Committee for Health Equity in ICD11 Borreliosis Codes. All Rights Reserved

[12] Balbus JA, Crimmins JL, Gamble DR, et al. (2016) Introduction: Climate change and human health. In: The impacts of climate change on human health in the united states: A scientific assessment, pp. 25-42, Washington, DC: U.S. Global Change Research Program.

[13] Boeckmann M and Joyner TA (2014) Old health risks in new places? An ecological niche model for I. ricinus tick distribution in Europe under a changing climate. Health & Place 30: 70-77.

[14] Brownstein JS, Holford TR, and Fish D (2005) Effect of climate change on Lyme disease risk in North America. EcoHealth 2(1): 38-46.

[15] DellaSala DA, Middelveen M, Liegner KB, Luche-Thayer J, Lyme Disease Epidemic Increasing Globally Due to Climate Change and Human Activities. Encyclopedia of the Anthropocene 2017 Elsevier Inc. http://dx.doi.org/10.1016/B978-0-12-409548-9.10516-0

[16] Gilbert L (2010) Altitudinal patterns of tick and host abundance: A potential role for climate change in regulating tick-borne diseases? Oecologia 162: 217e225.

[17] Korotkov Y, Kozlova T, and Kozlovskaya L (2015) Observations on changes in abundance of questing Ixodes ricinus, castor bean tick, over a 35-year period in the eastern part of its range (Russia, Tula region). Medical and Veterinary Entomology 29: 129-136.

[18] Medlock JM, Hansford KM, Bormane A, et al. (2013) Driving forces for changes in geographical distribution of Ixodes ricinus ticks in Europe. Parasites & Vectors 6: 1.

[19] Polgreen PM and Polgreen EL (2017) Emerging and re-emerging pathogens and diseases, and health consequences of a changing climate. In: Cohen J, Powderly WG, and Opal SM (eds.) Infectious diseases, 4th edn., pp. 40-48, Amsterdam: Elsevier. http://dx.doi.org/10.1016/B978-0-7020-6285-8.00004-6.

[20] Porretta D, Mastrantonio V, Amendolia S, et al. (2013) Effects of global changes on the climatic niche of the tick Ixodes ricinus inferred by species distribution modeling. Parasites and Vectors 6: 271.

[21] Simaon JA, Marrotte RR, Desrosiers N, et al. (2013) Climate change and habitat fragmentation drive the occurrence of Borrelia burgdorferi, the agent of Lyme disease, at the northeastern limit of its distribution. PLoS ONE 8(11), e80724.

[22] Sykes RA and Makiello P (2016) An estimate of Lyme borreliosis incidence in Western Europe. Journal of Public Health (Oxford, England). http://dx.doi.org/10.1093/pubmed/fdw017.

[23] The Ad Hoc Committee for Health Equity in ICD11 Borreliosis Codes' members represent highly skilled professionals from North and South America, Asia Pacific region, Africa, South America and Eastern, Western and Northern Europe. Many members are scientific and medical experts and have worked on borreliosis for two and three decades, and among them have many hundreds of peer-reviewed publications and studies. They serve as leaders, clinicians and professors across numerous well respected academic and research centers. The Ad Hoc Committee has members who consult regularly to the World Health

2

© Copyright 2018. Global Network on Institutional Discrimination and
Ad Hoc Committee for Health Equity in ICD11 Borreliosis Codes. All Rights Reserved

Organization (WHO) and governments on the development of health systems, surveillance practices, patient-centered care, ageing, zoonosis and other specialized areas. Other members are experts in law, governance, accountability, institutional reform, climate change, capacity building and human rights. The Ad Hoc Committee has members who have worked extensively with the private sector, from multinational corporations in multiple countries to local private education centers.

[24] O'Brien, JM, Hamidi OP (2017) Borreliosis Infection during Pregnancy, Ann Clin Cytol Pathol 3(8): 1085, www.jscimedcentral.com/ClinicalCytology/clinicalcytology-3-1085.pdf

[25] http://www.ohchr.org/EN/NewsEvents/Pages/DisplayNews.aspx?NewsID=21689

[26] The term Medically Unexplained Symptoms or MUS has been repudiated by the American Psychiatric Association (APA) and removed from the Diagnostic and Statistical Manual of Mental Disorders, 5th Edition or DSM-5.

[27] Sherr VT. Munchausen's syndrome by proxy and Lyme disease: medical misogyny or diagnostic mystery? Med Hypotheses. 2005;65(3):440-7 https://www.ncbi.nlm.nih.gov/pubmed/15925450

[28] Link to report from https://www.protecting-defenders.org/en/news/presentation-report-united-nations-general-assembly

[29] 2004 United Nations Convention against Corruption which followed the October 31, 2003 General Assembly resolution 58/4 to develop and support a comprehensive United Nations Convention against Corruption http://www.unodc.org/documents/treaties/UNCAC/Publications/Convention/08-50026_E.pdf

[30] September 1, 2016 Anti-Fraud and Anti-Corruption Framework for the United Nations Secretariat. http://www.un.org/es/ethics/pdf/anti_fraud_framework.pdf

[31] http://www.ohchr.org/Documents/Issues/MDGs/ Post2015/SDG_HR_Table.pdf.

[32] http://www.ohchr.org/ Documents/ Issues/ESCR/Health/ RightToHealthWHOFS2.pdf

[33] http://www.who.int/mediacentre/factsheets/fs323_en.pdf

[34] http://www.ifhhro.org/news-a-events/612-the-right-to-health-and-the-sustainable-development-goals]

[35] http://www.who.int/mediacentre/factsheets/fs323_en.pdf

[36] Open Society Institute and Equitas, "Appendix – Thirteen health and human rights documents," in Health and human rights: A resource guide (New York: Open Society Institute, 2007).

[37] Cohen J., Ezer T. Human rights in patient care: A theoretical and practical framework. Health and Human Rights Vol.15, No.2, Published December 10, 2013. https://sites.sph.harvard.edu/hhrjournal/2013/12/human-rights-in-patient-care-a-theoretical-and-practical-framework/ (This table is modified from original)

© Copyright 2018. Global Network on Institutional Discrimination and Ad Hoc Committee for Health Equity in ICD11 Borreliosis Codes. All Rights Reserved

[38]   Infectious diseases of the fetus and newborn infant, 6th Edition. Edited by Jack
        S Remington, Jerome O Klein, Christopher B Wilson, Carol J Baker. Published by
        Elsevier, Amsterdam, 2006, pp 1313. ISBN 0-7216-0537-0

[39]   Blood donor selection: guidelines on assessing donor suitability for blood
        donation. ISBN 978 92 4 154851 9 (NLM classification: WH 460) Development of
        this publication was supported by Cooperative Agreement Number PS024044
        from the United States Centers for Disease Control and Prevention (CDC). ©
        World Health Organization 2012 http://apps.who.int/iris/bitstream/10665/
        76724/1/9789241548519_eng.pdf

[40]   Infectious Diseases of the Fetus and Newborn Infant, 4th Edition. Edited by
        Jack S. Remington and Jerome O. Klein. 1373 pp., illustrated. Philadelphia,
        W.B. Saunders, 1995. ISBN: 0-7216-6782-1

[41]   Infectious Diseases of the Fetus and Newborn, 5th Edition Edited by Jack S.
        Remington and Jerome O. Klein Philadelphia: WB Saunders, 2001.

[42]   Peter Gøtzsche. Deadly Medicines and Organised Crime: How Big Pharma Has
        Corrupted Healthcare 1st Edition. Radcliffe Publishing LTD. St. Mark's House,
        Shepherdess Walk, London N17LH, United Kingdom. 2013. ISBN-13: 978-
        1846198847. ISBN-10: 1846198844

[43]   Johnson & Johnson to pay $2.2 billion to end U.S. drug probes by David Ingram
        and Ros Krasny. BUSINESS NEWS, November 4, 2013.
        https://www.reuters.com/article/us-jnj-settlement/johnson-johnson-to-pay-2-
        2-billion-to-end-u-s-drug-probes-idUSBRE9A30MM20131104

[44]   Corruption in the pharmaceutical sector, Diagnosing the challenges. Authors:
        Jillian Clare Kohler - Leslie Dan Faculty of Pharmacy, University of Toronto;
        WHO Collaborating Centre for Governance, Transparency & Accountability in
        the Pharmaceutical Sector. Martha Gabriela Martinez - Leslie Dan Faculty of
        Pharmacy, University of Toronto. Michael Petkov and James Sale –
        Transparency International,Pharmaceutical & Healthcare Programme. Design:
        Philip Jones – Transparency International UK. © 2016 Transparency
        International UK. All rights reserved

[45]   Cook M, Puri B. Commercial test kits for detection of Lyme borreliosis: A meta-
        analysis of test accuracy. International Journal of General Medicine. 2016;
        Volume 9:427-440. doi:10.2147/ijgm.s122313

[46]   Schwarzwalder A1, Schneider MF, Lydecker A, Aucott JN Sex differences in the
        clinical and serologic presentation of early Lyme disease: Results from a
        retrospective review. Gend Med. 2010 Aug;7(4):320-9. doi:
        10.1016/j.genm.2010.08.002

[47]   https://wonder.cdc.gov/wonder/prevguid/p0000380/p0000380.asp

[48]   Davidsson. M. The Financial Implications of a Well-Hidden and Ignored Chronic
        Lyme Disease Pandemic Healthcare 2018, 6(1), 16;
        doi:10.3390/healthcare6010016. Published: 13 February 2018.

[49]   John N. Aucott, Alison W. Rebman, Lauren A. Crowder, and Kathleen B. Kortte.
        Post-treatment Lyme disease syndrome symptomatology and the impact on life

4

© Copyright 2018. Global Network on Institutional Discrimination and
Ad Hoc Committee for Health Equity in ICD11 Borreliosis Codes. All Rights Reserved

functioning: is there something here? Qual Life Res. 2013 Feb; 22(1): 75-84. Published online 2012 Feb 1. doi: 10.1007/s11136-012-0126-6 PMCID: PMC3548099

[50]   Bransfield, R.C. Suicide and Lyme and associated diseases. Neuropsychiatr. Dis. Treat. 2017, 13, 1575-1587.

[51]   The incidence of Lyme disease in Europe was published in 2008 for the years 1996 to 2005 by the Health and Consumers Directorate-General of Directorate C Public Health and Risk Assessment and available at: http://ec.europa.eu/health//ph_information/dissemination/echi/docs/lyme_en.pdf

[52]   Muller I1, Freitag MH, Poggensee G, Scharnetzky E, Straube E, Schoerner Ch, Hlobil H, Hagedorn HJ, Stanek G, Schubert-Unkmeir A, Norris DE, Gensichen J, Hunfeld KP. Evaluating frequency, diagnostic quality, and cost of Lyme borreliosis testing in Germany: a retrospective model analysis. Clin Dev Immunol. 2012;2012:595427. doi: 10.1155/2012/595427. Epub 2011 Dec 27.

[53]   Felipe C. Cabello, Henry P. Godfrey, Julia V. Bugrysheva, Stuart A. Newman. Sleeper cells: the stringent response and persistence in the Borreliella (Borrelia) burgdorferi enzootic cycle. First published: 11 September 2017. DOI: 10.1111/1462-2920.13897. *Author Julia V. Bugrysheva works for the CDC and is affiliated with New York Medical College, Valhalla, NY, USA*

[54]   Zhang X, Meltzer MI, Peña CA, Hopkins AB, Wroth L, Fix AD. Economic Impact of Lyme Disease. Emerg Infect Dis. 2006 Apr; 12(4): 653–660. doi:10.3201/eid1204.050602 PMCID: PMC3294685. *Original 2006 study costs have been adjusted for inflation*

[55]   http://www.idsociety.org/Policy/

[56]   Assous MV. Textes d'experts - Méthodes du diagnostic biologique au cours des différentes manifestations de la borréliose de Lyme [Laboratory methods for the diagnosis of clinical forms of Lyme borreliosis] Médecine et maladies infectieuses 37 (2007) 487-495. Reçu et accepté le 15 janvier 2006. Publié par Elsevier Masson SAS. doi:10.1016/j.medmal.2006.01.019

[57]   www.aldf.com/pdf/ECCMID_Poster_4.22.10.pdf

[58]   Rebman AW, Soloski Aucott JM. Sex and Gender Impact Lyme Disease Immunopathology, Diagnosis and Treatment. Sex and Gender Differences in Infection and Treatments for Infectious Diseases pp 337-360.

[59]   Schwartzwalder A, Schneider MF, Lydecker A, and Aucott JN (2010) Brief report sex differences in the clinical and serologic presentation of early Lyme disease: Results from a retrospective review. Gender Medicine 7(4): 320-329.

[60]   Johan Bakken's recent publications include Auwaerter PG, Bakken JS, Dattwyler RJ, et al. Antiscience and ethical concerns associated with advocacy of Lyme disease, Lancet Infect Dis 2011;11(9):713-9

[61]   Perronne C. Lyme disease antiscience. Lancet Infect Dis. 2012; 12: 361-2. Doi: 10.1016/S1473-3099(12)70053-1

© Copyright 2018. Global Network on Institutional Discrimination and
Ad Hoc Committee for Health Equity in ICD11 Borreliosis Codes. All Rights Reserved

[62]   Stricker RB, Johnson L. Let's tackle the testing. Letter. 2007;335(7628):1008. doi:10.1136/bmj.39394. 676227.BE. http://dx.doi.org/10.1136/bmj.39394.676227.BE. Accessed February 19, 2017

[63]   Department of Health and Human Services' National Institutes of Health Response to the Conference Report Request for a Plan to Ensure Taxpayers' Interests are Protected. Page 7. July 2001. Web source: https://www.ott.nih.gov/sites/default/files/documents/policy/wydenrpt.Pdf Accessed 08.20.2017

[64]   http://www.idsociety.org/Policy/

[65]   IDSA Lyme Disease and State Policy Primer for State Legislators (Updated August 2016) http://www.idsociety.org/uploadedFiles/IDSA/Topics_of_ Interest/Lyme_Disease/Policy_Documents/Lyme%20state%20policy%20primer%2 0update%202016%20FINAL.pdf

[66]   Editors: Graham R, Mancher M, Wolman DM, Greenfield S, Steinberg E. Clinical Practice Guidelines We Can Trust. Institute of Medicine (US) Committee on Standards for Developing Trustworthy Clinical Practice Guidelines; Washington (DC): National Academies Press (US); 2011. Web Source: http://www.nationalacademies.

[67]   org/hmd/Reports/2011/Clinical-Practice-Guidelines-We-Can-Trust/Standards.aspx Accessed 01.20.2018

[68]   Schach Wendy H. The Bayh-Dole Act: Selected Issues in Patent Policy and the Commercialization of Technology. Congressional Research Service, December 3, 2012 https://fas.org/sgp/crs/misc/RL32076.pdf

[69]   Joseph G. Jemsek, MD, FACP, AAHIVS. 2007 White Paper for Connecticut Attorney General Richard Blumenthal on Conflicts of Interest in the 2006 'Clinical Assessment, Treatment, and Prevention of Lyme Disease, Human Granulocytic Anaplasmosis, and Babesiosis: Clinical Practice Guidelines by the Infectious Diseases Society of America'.

[70]   https://patents.justia.com/patent/7605248. Accessed February 27, 2018.

[71]   http://patft.uspto.gov/netacgi/nph-Parser?Sect1=PTO1&Sect2=HITOFF&d=PALL&p=1&u=%2Fnetahtml%2FPTO%2Fsrc hnum.htm&r=1&f=G&l=50&s1=4721617.PN.&OS=PN/4721617&RS=PN/4721617. Accessed 3.1.2018.

[72]   On November 10, 2017, a group of LB patients filed a federal antitrust lawsuit in the U.S. District Court for the Eastern District of Texas, Texarkana Division - Case 5:17-cv-00190-RWS. The patients allege that major health insurers are denying coverage for LB treatments based on "bogus" guidelines that were established by their paid consultants from the Infectious Diseases Society of America.

[73]   A Guide to the Rulemaking Process, Prepared by the Office of the Federal Register https://www.federalregister.gov/uploads/2011/01/the_rulemaking_ process.pdf

© Copyright 2018. Global Network on Institutional Discrimination and
Ad Hoc Committee for Health Equity in ICD11 Borreliosis Codes. All Rights Reserved

[74]   Email correspondence from 'Highlights CDC FOIAs Kris Newby'. HB 836 required the Maryland's Secretary of Health and Mental Hygiene, in collaboration with other State agencies, to establish and promote a public awareness campaign for the prevention of Lyme and other tick-borne diseases.

Johnson, Barbara J. (CDC/CCID/NCZVED)

From: Johnson, Barbara J. (CDC/CCID/NCZVED)
Sent: Wednesday, March 28. 2007 9:03AM
To: 'Edward McSweegan'
Cc: Mead, Paul
Subject: RE: Maryland Lyme Disease Public Awareness Bill (HB 838)

David Blythe
State Epidemiologist xxx-xxx-xxxx

Ed,

This is the contact information for the state epidemiologist. Paul, is this current? If not, please send us both a link to the list of all the state epis.

Barbara

From: Edward McSweegan
Sent: Wednesday, March 28, 2007 8:05 AM .
To: Wormser, Gary; 'Leasure, Mark'; 'Olson, Diana'; 'Durland Fish'; 'Linda Bockenstedt'; 'steve dumler'; 'allen steere'; Johnson, Barbara J. (COC/CCID/NCZVED); 'eugene shapiro'; 'franc strle'; 'gerold stanek'; 'johan bakken'; john halperln'; 'mark klempner'; Mead, Paul (CDC/CCID/NCZVED); 'peter krause'; 'ray dattwyler'; 'robert nadelman'; volker fingerle'; 'arthur weinstein'; Johnson, Barbara J. (CDC/CCID/NCZVED); 'bettlna wilske'; 'donna mckenna'; 'hank feder'; 'harvey artsob'; 'ira schwartz'; 'jerry green'; 'john nowakowski'; 'Munoz, Jose'; 'Juan Salazar'; 'Justin Radolf'; 'Lawrence Zemel'; 'maria aguero'; 'muhammad morshed'; 'paul auwaerter'; 'Richand Porwancher'; 'robert smith'; 'Rosalie Trevejo'; 'sue o'connell'; 'sunil sood'; 'susan wong'; 'tom draper'; Phillip Baker
Subject: Maryland;Lyme Public Awareness Bill (HB 836)

Anyone have any contacts in the Maryland Dept. of Health who would be interested in knowing about this Maryland bill and the efforts of activists to kill it?

ed

---

[75]   http://www.ohchr.org/EN/Issues/SRHRDefenders/Pages/Challenges.aspx
[76]   Government of Denmark's TV2's documentary 'Cheating or Borrelia'
[77]   Wormser GP, Shapiro ED. Implications of Gender in Chronic Lyme Disease. Womens Health (Larchmt). 2009 Jun; 18(6): 831–834. doi: 10.1089/jwh.2008.1193 PMCID: PMC2913779
[78]   http://www.idsociety.org/IDSA_Statement_on_Reintroduction_of_Home_Infusion_Legislation/
[79]   Infection Lapses Rampant In Nursing Homes But Punishment Is Rare
https://www.washingtonpost.com/national/health-science/infection-lapses-rampant-in-nursing-homes-but-punishment-is-rare/2017/12/22/0d6c61bc-e701-11e7-927a-e72eac1e73b6_story.html?utm_term=.c6e2a80d7b6d
[80]   Salzman MB1, Rubin LG. Vascular catheter-related infection is an important cause of mortality and morbidity in hospitalized patients. Adv Pediatr Infect Dis. 1995;10:337-68. Intravenous catheter-related infections. Department of Pediatrics, Kaiser Foundation Hospital-West Los Angeles, California, USA. https://www.ncbi.nlm.nih.gov/pubmed/7718211

© Copyright 2018. Global Network on Institutional Discrimination and
Ad Hoc Committee for Health Equity in ICD11 Borreliosis Codes. All Rights Reserved

[81] Cheung E, Baerlocher MO, Asch M, Myers A. Venous access, A practical review for 2009. Can Fam Physician. 2009 May; 55(5): 494-496. PMCID: PMC2682308 https://www.ncbi.nlm.nih.gov/pmc/articles/PMC2682308/

[82] Farm antibiotic use in the United States August 2017. Alliance to Save our Antibiotics. http://www.saveourantibiotics.org/media/1773/farm-antibiotic-use-in-the-united-states.pdf

[83] Availability, Accessibility, Acceptability, Quality (AAAQ) of care 1136/bmj.39394. 676227.BE. http://dx.doi.org/10.1136/bmj.39394.676227.BE. Accessed February 19, 2017

[84] http://www.ohchr.org/Documents/Publications/Factsheet31.pdf http://www.ohchr.org/Documents/Issues/ESCR/Health/RightToHealthWHOFS2

[85] https://www.canlii.org/en/on/onhparb/doc/2013/2013canlii68994/2013canlii68994.html?searchUrlHash=AAAAAQAEbHltZQAAAAAB&resultIndex=3

[86] https://techmedweb.omb.state.or.us/Clients/ORMB/Public/VerificationDetails.aspx?EntityID=1461213

[87] http://www.cvbd.org/en/tick-borne-diseases/lyme-borreliosis/distribution/

[88] Feder, Henry M. et al. 2007. "A Critical Appraisal of Chronic Lyme Disease." New England Journal of Medicine 357(14):1422-30. (http://www.nejm.org/doi/abs/10.1056/NEJMra072023).

[89] Wormser GP, Dattwyler RJ, Shapiro ED, Halperin JJ,3, Steere AC, Klempner MS, Krause PJ, Bakken JS, Strle F, Stanek G, Bockenstedt L, Fish D, Dumler S, Nadelman RB. The Clinical Assessment, Treatment, and Prevention of Lyme Disease, Human Granulocytic Anaplasmosis, and Babesiosis: Clinical Practice Guidelines by the Infectious Diseases Society of America. Clinical Infectious Diseases 2006; 43:1089-134. 2006 by the Infectious Diseases Society of America. All rights reserved. 1058-4838/2006/4309-0001. http://www.idsociety.org/uploadedFiles/IDSA/Guidelines-Patient_Care/PDF_Library/Lyme%20Disease.pdf

[90] Much of this information comes from an interview by Huib Kraaijeveld, MA in Social Psychology. Kraaijeveld is a LB advocate, researcher and author, with extensive experience in international business and leadership education and professional service firms at Nyenrode Business University. As chairman of the On Lyme Foundation, he has been building bridges between different groups of knowledge owners in the field of medical expertise, as well as the many social, bureaucratic, financial and legal areas challenging those living with LB and co-infections. Kraaijeveld authored Shifting the Lyme Paradigm; a Caretakers Guide on a Heroes Journey.

[91] Sin Hang Lee, Veronica S Vigliotti, Jessica S Vigliotti, Suri Pappu. Routine human papillomavirus genotyping by DNA sequencing in community hospital laboratories. Infect Agent Cancer. 2007; 2: 11. Published online 2007 Jun 5. doi: 10.1186/1750-9378-2-1. PMCID: PMC1894957 https://www.ncbi.nlm.nih.gov/pmc/articles/PMC1894957/

8

© Copyright 2018. Global Network on Institutional Discrimination and
Ad Hoc Committee for Health Equity in ICD11 Borreliosis Codes. All Rights Reserved

[92] https://www.canada.ca/en/public-health/services/laboratory-biosafety-biosecurity/pathogen-safety-data-sheets-risk-assessment/rickettsia-rickettsii.html

[93] https://www.canada.ca/en/public-health/services/laboratory-biosafety-biosecurity/pathogen-safety-data-sheets-risk-assessment/rickettsia-rickettsii.html

[94] Sciences et Avenir article "Lyme disease could be a new health scandal in France" https://www.sciencesetavenir.fr/sante/alain-trautmann-la-maladie-de-lyme-pourrait-etre-un-nouveau-scandale-sanitaire-en-france_118731

[95] BC doctor urged to retire because of zealous approach to Lyme disease. Kathy Tomlinson, CBC News Posted: Nov 18, 2008 7:26 AM PT Last Updated: Nov 18, 2008 7:19 AM PT. http://www.cbc.ca/news/canada/british-columbia/b-c-doctor-urged-to-retire-because-of-zealous-approach-to-lyme-disease-1.774679

[96] Press release of October 26, 2017: The Academy of Medicine denounces deceptions about Lyme disease. Posted on October 26, 2017 http://www.academie-medecine.fr/communique-de-presse-du-26102017-lacademie-de-medecine-denonce-les-tromperies-a-propos-de-la-maladie-de-lyme/

[97] Robert Alexander Sykes RA. An Estimate of Lyme Borreliosis Incidence in Western Europe. Journal of the Royal Medical Society. Vol. 22 No. 1: Winter 2014/ Clinical Review Article

[98] Pfeiffer MB. Swedish MD suspended over Lyme disease care; patients bereft https://www.huffingtonpost.com/entry/swedish-md-suspended-over- lyme-disease-care-patients_us_58b9e03de4b02b8b584dfb74

[99] https://www.wma.net/policies-post/wma-declaration-of-helsinki-ethical-principles-for-medical-research-involving-human-subjects/

[100] Øines Ø, Radzijevskaja J, Paulauskas A, Rosef O. Prevalence and diversity of Babesia spp. in questing Ixodes ricinusticks from Norway. Parasit Vectors. 2012; 5: 156. Published online 2012 Aug 4. doi: 10.1186/1756-3305-5-156 PMCID: PMC3439691

[101] Lyme patient receives compensation 10 years after inadequate treatment. https://www.aftenposten.no/norge/i/rLWWB0/Borreliosepasient-far-erstatning-10-ar-etter-manglende-behandling. Published: 05 JAN, 2018: 05:51 English translation by Angelica Johansson VIDAS ©.

[102] Morten M. Laane, Ivar Mysterud. A simple method for the detection of live Borrelia spirochaetes in human blood using classical microscopy techniques. Biological and Biomedical Reports, 2013, 3(1), 15-28 http://counsellingme.com/microscopy/MysterudAndLaane.pdf

[103] Sustainable Governance Indicators (SGI) - 2015 Denmark Report- Finn Laursen, Torben M. Andersen, Detlef Jahn (Coordinator) http://www.sgi-network.org/docs/2015/country/SGI2015_Denmark.pdf

[104] https://www.sst.dk/da/rationel-farmakoterapi/maanedsbladet/2010/maanedsblad_nr_7_juli_2010/borreliose

© Copyright 2018. Global Network on Institutional Discrimination and Ad Hoc Committee for Health Equity in ICD11 Borreliosis Codes. All Rights Reserved

[105] Dessau RB, Espenhain L, Mølbak K, Krause TG, Voldstedlund M. Improving national surveillance of Lyme neuroborreliosis in Denmark through electronic reporting of specific antibody index testing from 2010 to 2012. (PMID:26212143) Euro Surveillance : Bulletin Europeen sur les Maladies Transmissibles = European Communicable Disease Bulletin [16 Jul 2015, 20(28)] https://www.ncbi.nlm.nih.gov/pubmed/26212143

[106] Harvey, WT, Martz, D. Motor neuron disease recovery associated with IV ceftriaxone and anti-Babesia therapy. Acta Neurologica Scandinavica. Volume 115 Issue – 2. 2007. Blackwell Publishing Ltd. UR - http://dx.doi.org/10.1111/j.1600-0404.2006.00727.x .

[107] https://www.nysenate.gov/newsroom/articles/kathleen-marchione/dr-kari-w-bovenzi

[108] Amid medical controversy, children saved. By T Stephenson. April 5, 2011. https://yaledailynews.com/blog/2011/04/05/amid-medical-controversy-children-saved/disease

[109] https://archive.org/details/lymediseasediagn00unit

[110] Report to the UN General Assembly 30 July 30, 2015 by SR Michel Forst https://www.protecting-defenders.org/pdf.js/web/viewer.html?file=https%3A//www.protecting-defenders.org/sites/protecting-defenders.org/files/A-70-217-ENG_1.pdf

[111] www.ifhhro.org/ news-a-events/612-the-right-to-health-and-the-sustainable-development-goals

[112] http://www.independent.co.uk/news/uk/home-news/un-disabled-rights-uk-government-denounced-criticised-united-nations-austerity-policies-a7923006.html

[113] http://www.independent.co.uk/voices/disability-cuts-department-for-work-and-pensions-esa-a7560961.html

[114] https://twitter.com/lymemoms/status/970017986781233152
https://twitter.com/MoriartyLab/status/970038162553651200
https://twitter.com/MoriartyLab/status/970044897876049920

[115] http://www.virology.ws/2016/02/10/open-letter-lancet-again/

[116] David F Marks. Special issue on the PACE Trial. Journal of Health Psychology. July 31, 2017. http://journals.sagepub.com/doi/full/10.1177/1359105317722370

[117] PACE Trail Debate on behalf of the Myalgic Encephalomyelitis Community Feb. 20, 2018. Glasgow MP Carol Monaghan leads a debate about the controversial flawed PACE Trial upon those living with Myalgic Encephalomyelitis (ME/CFS) in the UK and worldwide. https://www.youtube.com/watch?v=UwCEvnXZTlA&feature=youtu.be

10

© Copyright 2018. Global Network on Institutional Discrimination and
Ad Hoc Committee for Health Equity in ICD11 Borreliosis Codes. All Rights Reserved

www.ingramcontent.com/pod-product-compliance
Lightning Source LLC
Chambersburg PA
CBHW081731220526

45468CB00008B/2062